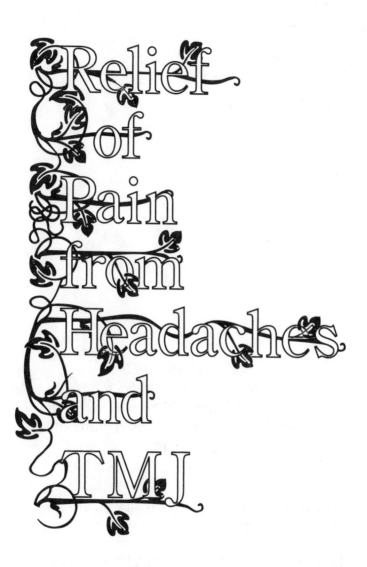

Relief of Pain from Headaches and TMJ

Paula Mackowiak, M.S. P.T.
Physical Therapist

Medical illustrations by Steven Moskowitz
Cover design and art by Michael Chapman

PRINTED IN THE UNITED STATES OF AMERICA
Manhattan Printing
3095 Elmwood Avenue
Buffalo, New York 14217

Paula Mackowiak was awarded her Bachelor of Science Degree in the field of physical therapy from the University of Florida. She received her Master of Science Degree from the Medical College of Virginia.

Contents

To my family who got me started.

To my patients who keep me going.

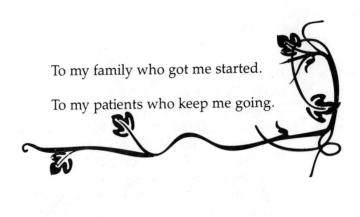

Opening Comments

This book is about headaches, and about the temporomandibular joint (TMJ). If you are experiencing headaches, your jaw joint may or may not be a contributing factor. Likewise, if you are experiencing a jaw problem, you may or may not be having headaches. A large part of this book focuses on the TMJ, and the role it plays in the production of all kinds of pain. Another large part of this book focuses on headaches in general.

Technical terms are boldfaced in the text and defined in the glossary, located in the Resource Section.

Acknowledgements

For every line that appears written in a book, scores have passed before. Writing is the most painstaking and the most exhilarating work there is. I now know why Hemingway said when asked how to write a book, "First you clean the refrigerator." I also know why van Gogh cut off his ear. Writers are artists who use words as their medium. They are a subculture of society who sit over pad and keys awaiting the breathing in of inspiration; desiring to share, enlighten, and learn. The people who helped me keep both ears during the writing of this manuscript are: Kate Grimes, Meryl Cohen, Mary Mackowiak, Claudia Griffith, Genie Foreman, and Jerry Cone for their unending emotional support, Steven Moskowitz, who drew and created many of the beautiful medical illustrations, Mike and Sam Solomon, who offered their brilliant guiding light, Sister Mary Jerome, who enlivened the writing process within me, and whose spirit lives in the writing, and the Creator, from whom all things are created. And to all of my patients who continue to teach me a better way, I thank you.

Prologue

Understanding is the ultimate empowerment tool. When you understand something the mystique is removed, the confusion lifts and the mind can think clearly. Understanding is also the ultimate seduction of the mind. When we discover something about ourselves it satisfies a place very deep within us. That discovery goes beyond words and changes us forever.

This book is a tool. The facts that are presented about headaches and Temporomandibular Joint Syndrome (TMJ) will dispel the myths and lift the confusion, so that you can become part of the solution. How you use it and how powerful you become depends on you. TMJ is not something that has been inflicted on you that will be removed by someone for a fee. TMJ is an experience that you have helped to create. Now you can help dissolve it by being open to discovery about yourself, and by knowing that you can create for yourself your own level of well being.

Arm yourself with the facts. By gathering them you will begin to gain an understanding of the limits and possibilities. Then take the leap of faith that you will be well again. Trust yourself. You know the answers already.

Introduction

e seek not rest, but transformation.
We are dancing through each other
as doorways.

— Marge Piercy

One

Anyone who has experienced locking of their jaw, or sharp sudden jaw pain has had an experience unequaled. The medical maze through which these people pass is equally unequaled. After **CT scans**, drugs, and numerous doctor/therapy appointments, often they remain without answers or relief.

If you are one of the lucky ones, you were referred to a dentist who has been competently trained to treat TMJ. TMJ, as it is commonly called, stands for temporomandibular joint dysfunction which is primarily a jaw disorder that can give rise to numerous symptoms. The most common of these symptoms is pain in the jaw, ear, head and neck. It is often accompanied by stiffness, locking, and/or clicking of the jaw joint. TMJ is one of the most difficult conditions to diagnose because often there is no **organic disease** in the joint itself. The symptoms mimic other conditions, and pain is commonly referred to the jaw from the neck area. Even though this is a complex condition and a relatively new area to be addressed in the fields of medicine and dentistry, there are practitioners who are treating TMJ effectively. It is of utmost importance that you find these practitioners and begin to develop a working relationship with them.

It is conservatively estimated that 10 million people in this country have TMJ. Although a large majority (75%) of them are women between the ages of 20-50, there has been an increase in the incidence among men and children. A leading specialist in the area of TMJ, Dr. Harold Gelb, proposes that this condition is a primary initiating factor in 80% of all **chronic** pain disorders, and that one third of the population presently has some medical condition which is aggravated by a jaw imbalance. For a society which spends an estimated $25 billion on drugs, surgeries, and psychotherapy, the implications of Dr. Gelb's statement are far reaching. What he is suggesting is that TMJ may be an underlying cause of many of the chronic pain conditions that are so prevalent today such as low back pain and headaches. This is a strong statement by Dr. Gelb, and one which requires further examination.

Because TMJ is difficult to diagnose, and because the variety of symptoms are so varied, (over 100 documented complaints), this condition has become the new "dumping" diagnosis. If a specific diagnosis cannot be made for your condition, you may be dumped into the category TMJ. It is now fashionable and trendy to have TMJ. The old trends were sciatica for back and leg pain and thoracic outlet syndrome for neck and arm pain. THESE ARE NOT DIAGNOSES! They merely label the part of the body with the symptom.

All pain down the leg is not caused by pressure on the sciatic nerve. All pain down the arm is not caused by pressure on the nerves that go into the arm. And all face pain is not caused by the jaw joint. There is now strong data by many respected researchers which shows that any structure that has a nerve going to it can cause referred pain, i.e. pain down an arm or a leg, or into the jaw area. That means that the muscles, ligaments, or any structure which has a nerve supply, join in to complicate matters, but also help us to make a more definitive diagnosis. The practitioners you seek help from will determine the underlying contributing factors which are causing your pain, whether that be the way in which your teeth meet, your muscles, your posture, or your lifestyle.

And those people who have suffered with headaches know the frustration of being told, after being subjected to test after test, that all of the findings were negative, that they have headaches or migraines, and that they have to learn to live with the problem. What is the current offering to many of these individuals is a lifetime of medication, suggestions for dietary changes, relaxation exercises, and the hope that at menopause the headaches will subside. If you are a man, the last one is of no consolation at all. And if you are a thirty year old woman, twenty years is a long time to wait. A better solution is needed, and this book offers that solution.

The information in this book will be limited to the discussion of chronic pain conditions where there has not been major trauma to the jaw or head, and where there is an absence of disease. In other words, we will be dealing with **dysfunction** not disease. Most people do not have tumors or fractures of their jaw or skull. Those who do, need close medical supervision which is beyond the scope of this book. The very large majority of people with TMJ and headaches do have a **dysfunction** in one or more areas that will be presented in much detail. Some of these **dysfunctions** include a change in the way the teeth meet, a mechanical problem in the joint, a change in the posture, muscle imbalances, and the development of poor habits, such as clenching and grinding. A whole host of changes occur in the body when these situations arise, which have profound effects on the entire body.

We don't have absolutes. This area is not like other areas of medicine that are based on more scientific evidence. Henceforth, you will come across individuals who don't believe in TMJ, who dismiss it as a condition. And there are many who pass off headaches as stress related. Presently, no research has been completed that definitively <u>proves</u> that treatments have an effect. This merely suggests that we should progress onward in the way that we evaluate and treat headaches and TMJ, without claiming absolutes, but by using educated analyses, common sense, and past clinical experience as guideposts. TMJ is real. Headaches are real. They do exist, and often have a structural basis. People are being helped every day by competently trained professionals who are familiar with treating these areas.

The onus is on our professions to substantiate our claims, and we will. This is a new area, and we are just now observing the connections between the objective signs that we see, and correlating them with the symptoms. Observation always precedes testing. Even the strongest research, when applied without common sense or good clinical judgement, is not useful. For example, a dislocated **disc** of the right TMJ causing right TMJ pain can be a poor correlation for that person when they wake up after surgery with the same face pain. The findings from the most impressive research must still be applied clinically, to you, the intricate unique human being that you are. More on this later...

People often come to my clinic who have been to doctors and dentists who have told them that they have to live with the pain and to see a psychiatrist. I continue to be astounded. When a person is in distress, it is not helpful to suggest that there is no hope to ever get rid of the pain and that they are making it up, which is how the patient interprets this advice. My advice is to be wary of anyone who destroys hope! The state of the art in medicine is that hope and belief are probably THE deciding factors in favor of the patient recovering. Dr. Siegel, in his book Love Medicine and Miracles, talks about these factors.

Take for example two people given the same diagnosis of Cancer. One accepts it as a death sentence and dies. The other one defies the odds and lives. A miracle is possible. The will to live is probable. The will to get better wins. A healthy realism is important. Just be very protective of who or what you let influence that inner part of you which is the hope and dream of you being well again.

In the past several years I have to admit that this archaic way of treating an individual in distress is becoming less. I want to believe it is because doctors are changing their attitudes. Another factor is that patients are taking matters into their own hands and finding legitimate alternatives that work for them, unfortunately without their physician's blessing. I say unfortunately because both the physician and the patient lose as a result of this breakdown in communication. Patients begin to sense early on how much input they are going to have in the decision making process. Open lines of communication are healthy and necessary to preserve the physician-patient bond. What you can do about it is to choose a doctor that is open to alternative methods of treatment but who will remain the overall coordinator of your care.

Some of the information in this book you need to know, and some of it is nice to know. If there is a trend in my practice it is that people want to know....lots. I include more than you need to know. A great thespian once said to me, "You have to go overboard to be on-board." I believed it then for work in the theater and I believe it now for writing.

THEORIES ABOUT TMJ

The most common cause of TMJ is proposed by some dentists to be the improper position of the jaw **(mandible)** caused by improper position of the teeth **(malocclusion)**. Another popular view is proposed to be that a **malocclusion** alters the position of the jaw joint and strains the muscles, which leads to an abnormal feeling or sensation in the jaw area. This abnormal sensation can then cause

muscle spasm and pain. Also identified as a cause of TMJ is muscle fatigue that develops as a result of clenching and/or grinding behavior. Muscle fatigue can lead to **muscle spasm** and pain. This is referred to as **myofascial pain dysfunction (MPD)**, and is generally accepted now as the leading cause of TMJ. It appears as if philosophically dentists are moving away from identifying **occlusion** as the primary cause and are moving toward a muscle based theory as the primary cause of TMJ.

In the profession of physical therapy, we also view the primary cause of TMJ to be **myofascial**, and take the explanation one step further. The TMJ is viewed in relation to the whole body. When observed in relation to the whole, the TMJ becomes an extension of the spine, dependent on the functioning of the entire mechanical structure. As musculoskeletal imbalances begin to occur throughout the body, the jaw, being dependent upon a balanced spine, is just the final victim at the end of a long **kinetic chain**. A balanced spine means one which is strong, flexible, and straight. Alter the supporting structure for the jaw, and the stage is set for a variety of possibilities such as **muscle spasm** and pain. I will explain this fully at a later time.

Probably the real truth is that the cause of TMJ includes a combination of all the different theories. This book is not meant to be a contest between who is right, dentists or physical therapists. What physical therapists are coming to recognize is the importance of dental input in relation to proper support of the jaw from the teeth. What dentists are beginning to recognize is the importance of input from other health professionals in treating the musculoskeletal system. And what we are all recognizing is the importance of the **myofascial** system as it relates to TMJ and headache. This is an area where cliche or no cliche we have to work together.

When asked what a physical therapist does, most people would respond that they teach people how to walk with crutches, exercise weak limbs, or apply heat treatments to a back. While that may still be true, the profession has shown enormous growth, particularly in the area of orthopedics, which includes TMJ. The level of sophistication in evaluation and treatment techniques is high. Many physical therapists are now well educated in mechanics of the spine, **craniosacral therapy**, **myofascial release**, use of high technology modalities such as **laser**, high frequency **electrical stimulation**, and **acupuncture point** stimulation. Since physical therapists have been treating the musculoskeletal system for over 50 years and as we move toward a muscle based theory as to the cause of TMJ, I am proposing that with our background, physical therapists are the most qualified individuals to treat the muscular component of this problem. Many physicians and dentists have already come to rely heavily on these clinicians in the overall management of their chronic pain cases. FIND THESE PEOPLE!

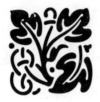

How

The

Jaw

Functions

e shall not cease from exploration.
And at the end of all our exploring
Will be to arrive from where we started
And know the place for the first time.
— T.S. Eliot

𝕿wo

We use our jaw joints an estimated 1500-2000 times per day during the activities of chewing, swallowing, talking, yawning and sneezing. The movements that are allowed at the TMJ are opening, closing, forward and backward glide, and lateral, or side glide. See Figures 1,2, and 3.

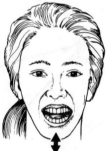

Figure 1. Opening and
closing motions.

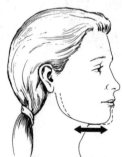

Figure 2. Forward and backward
glide motions.

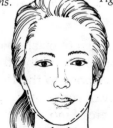

Figure 3. Side glide motions.

Normal opening is considered to be the ability to place your index, middle and ring fingers between the top and bottom teeth. See Figure 4.

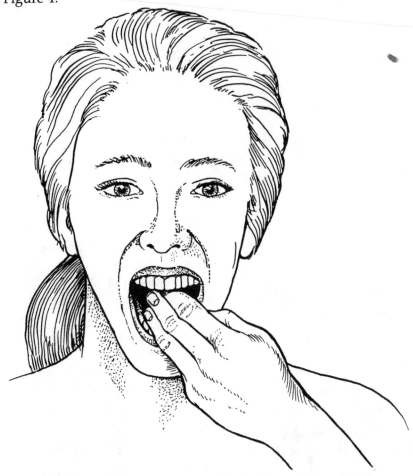

Figure 4. Normal opening is present when the index, middle, and ring fingers can be inserted between the front teeth.

The quality of the opening motion should be such that there is no joint noise (clicking or popping) and that the jaw opens in a smooth straight line, with no deviations to the right or left. See Figures 5 and 6. To check the quality of your opening motion stand in front of a mirror and observe the arc of motion your jaw moves through as you open and close. Are your top and bottom teeth lined up when your jaw is closed? Does your jaw stay aligned when you open?

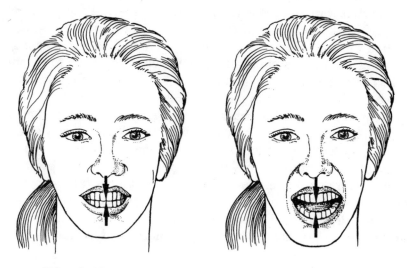

Figure 5. *Normal mandibular alignment and normal mandibular motion.*

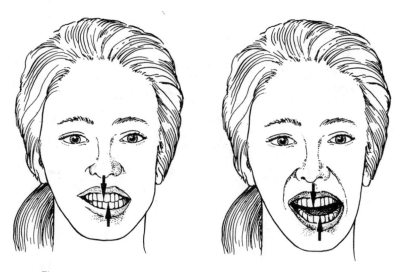

Figure 6. *Asmymmetrical mandibular alignment and abnormal mandibular motion.*

Closing should similarly be smooth and quiet, and follow a straight line. Lateral glide should be equal to both sides. There is more forward glide than backward glide. During forward glide the bottom teeth should be able to move just forward of the top teeth. Check yourself in the mirror to see if your lateral or side motion is equal and forward glide is normal. NORMAL RANGE OF MOTION IS NECESSARY FOR THE JOINT TO FUNCTION PROPERLY.

When the jaw is at rest, i.e. when you are not talking or eating, the tip of the tongue should be positioned behind the top front teeth. This is the same position that the tongue is in when you say the word, "in." The rest of the tongue is held onto the roof of the mouth by suction. This normal resting position of the tongue forces the teeth to separate slightly creating what is called a **freeway space** between the teeth. You should feel that the jaw is in its most relaxed position here, although it may feel different if this is a new position for you. You should be able to breath comfortably through your nose with your tongue in this position. Many people allow their tongues to drop to the floor of the mouth. This position is incorrect. Normal resting position of the tongue is illustrated in Figure 7.

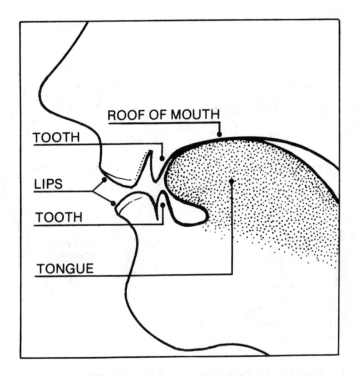

Figure 7. Normal resting position of the tongue is achieved when the tip of the tongue maintains light contact with the top front teeth. When the tongue is in this position, the jaw is in its most relaxed state.

The TMJ is now in its resting position which is a non-weightbearing position. Although the jaw is designed for powerful clenching and the teeth are durable structures, the area is not designed for prolonged weight bearing. Gum chewing, eraser or pencil chewing, and clenching and grinding behavior, which is referred to as **bruxism,** all place undue stress on the area. People who breathe with their mouths open out of habit, or because of closed nasal passages, alter the normal functioning of this area. This needs correction.

The TMJ is shaped anatomically like a ball and socket joint. However, it is considered a **hinge joint** because its primary function is opening and closing, just as the hinges on a door allow for opening and closing. Side glide or lateral glide is considered an important accessory motion. Between the **condyle** (ball) of the **mandible** (jaw) and the **fossa** (socket) of the **temporal bone** lies a **disc** made of **cartilage** that is attached in front of the joint to a muscle called the **lateral pterygoid**. See Figure 8.

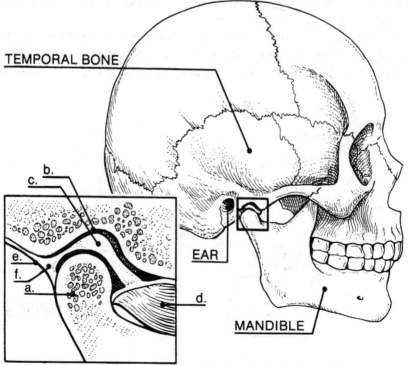

Figure 8. Anatomy of the TMJ. a. mandibular condyle, b. mandibular fossa, c. disc, d. lateral ptygeroid muscle, e. joint capsule, f. posterior ligament.

Also in Figure 8 notice how very close the joint lies to the ear. Through this anatomical closeness and shared nerve pathways, abnormalities in the joint often give rise to ear symptoms, the most common being pain, fullness, and ringing. Ringing of the ears is referred to as **tinnitis**. Other sensations my patients have reported to me are itchiness, wetness, a warm or cool sensation, and sounds other than ringing.

Crepitus is a term used to describe joint noise. It is characterized by crackling sounds in a joint upon motion. This occurs when there is roughening of the contacting surfaces of a joint. The most common cause of **crepitus** is osteoarthritis, which is simply degeneration of a joint. As the **cartilage** which covers bone begins to wear, bone meets bone at the joint surfaces. This is not as good a contacting surface as **cartilage** on bone, or **cartilage** on **cartilage**. Hence, you can get joint noise. A certain amount of joint noise is considered acceptable in all joints. **Tendons**, **ligaments**, and **discs** can reorient themselves upon movement, causing some joint noise. However, when it becomes excessive or when it is accompanied by pain, it is considered abnormal.

Opening the jaw requires a complex motion of the joint where the **condyle** of the **mandible** rolls on the **disc** and the **disc** glides forward in the **fossa** of the **temporal bone**. See Figures 9 and 10.

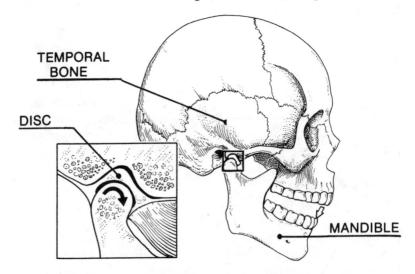

TEMPORAL BONE

DISC

MANDIBLE

Figure 9. In the early phase of opening, the condyle (ball) rolls in place on the disc. This mechanical action of rolling is what allows for opening of the jaw.

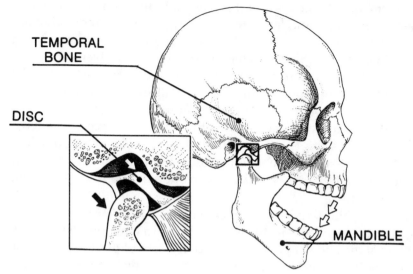

TEMPORAL BONE

DISC

MANDIBLE

Figure 10. In the latter phase of opening, the disc glides forward in the fossa. This mechanical action of gliding results in the full opening of the jaw.

Gravity and relaxation of the closing muscles begins the opening motion. One portion of the **lateral pterygoid muscle** pulls on the **mandible** to open the jaw while another portion of the muscle glides the **disc** forward in the **fossa** of the **temporal bone**. This **rolling** motion first and **gliding** motion later in the range of motion are extremely important components of opening motion.

A **ligament** in the posterior compartment of the joint limits the forward motion of the **disc** on full opening. See Figure 8. If this **ligament** becomes torn, which often occurs during **whiplash** of the neck, or irritated, as a result of holding the mouth open too long during a dental procedure, normal joint mechanics can be disrupted.

The joint **capsule** is a structure composed of thick **connective tissue** which surrounds and supports the entire joint. The joint **capsule** is illustrated in Figure 8, but only the posterior portion is drawn. Anyone who has tried to separate a chicken leg from a thigh has experienced the strength of a joint **capsule**. The tautness or looseness of the **capsule** greatly determines the amount of opening motion allowed at the joint. If one part of the **capsule** becomes tight it can cause limited opening and deviation to the side that is tight.

The **mandible** moves as if it is one joint but it is a paired joint in that it has a right and left side. In no other place in the body does this occur. Motion is dependent on freedom of movement and coordination of both sides. If one side develops a problem, the other side automatically compensates. For example in Figure 6, if the left joint **capsule** becomes tight the jaw will deviate to the left on opening. Thus, pain could be experienced on the left side. But it is also possible to experience pain on the right side since deviation to the left strains the tissues on the right side. The actual problem could be present on the side opposite the pain. Therefore, even though symptoms are experienced on one side, both sides must be evaluated fully.

Opening the jaw is a complex movement. First, the posterior **ligament** must allow the **disc** to move forward while also limiting its motion at the end of opening. Second, the **lateral pterygoid muscle** must contract asynchronously. This means that one part of the muscle moves the **condyle** of the **mandible** on the **disc**, and another part of the muscle moves the **disc** in the **fossa**. Third, the joint **capsule** must allow movement while limiting the extremes of movement. Fourth, the joint space must be free of debris and swelling.

Synovial fluid is the lubrication inside the joint that provides a frictionless surface. Researchers have not been able to reproduce anything close to it in the laboratory (it's **coefficient of friction** is .001, which means it is very slick). The **synovial membrane**, which lines the joint, produces **synovial fluid**. If this membrane becomes irritated either by small stresses over a long time or by trauma to the joint, it can begin to produce too much fluid or a more **viscous** fluid. This leads to joint swelling and stiffness. Only a very small amount of this incredibly slick substance is present in the joint, but its contribution to smooth, effortless motion is great.

During closing of the jaw, the **disc** glides backward on the **temporal bone** and the **condyle** rolls back on the **disc**. Closing of the jaw is performed by the **temporalis, masseter,** and **medial pterygoid** muscles. These muscles have excellent leverage. Therefore, the motion of closing can be quite forceful. Figure 11 shows the anatomical placement of these muscles. In addition, you can feel these muscles on yourself. Place your fingers on your temples and clench your jaw. The muscle contracting under your fingers is called the **temporalis muscle**. Now place your fingers on your cheeks and clench. The muscle contracting under your fingers is the **masseter** and under the **masseter** is the **medial pterygoid**.

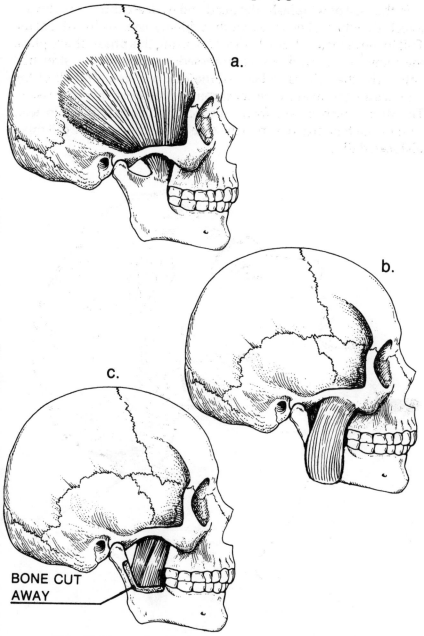

Figure 11. *The muscles of closing. a. temporalis, b. masseter, c. medial ptygeroid.*

SITUATIONS WHICH ALTER NORMAL FUNCTIONING

In the case of **whiplash**, the head and neck are thrown backward forcefully, which opens the mouth suddenly, causing the **disc** of the TMJ to move forward. See Figure 12. During this phase of **whiplash** the joints of the neck are compressed posteriorly and stretched anteriorly, the tissues in back of the **disc** are torn, and all of the muscles are traumatized either through stretching or compression. The **disc**, which moves forward quickly and forcefully, can tear, shift too far forward, or slip to the side off the **condyle**. We call this a **dislocated disc**.

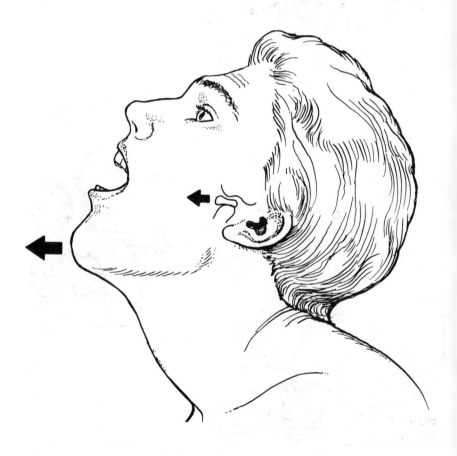

Figure 12. The hyperextension phase of whiplash. The arrows indicate force.

The second phase of **whiplash** is shown in Figure 13. The head is thrown forward forcefully, which stretches the posterior neck tissues. The neck is compressed anteriorly and the jaw is jammed closed. The tissues behind the **disc** get compressed from the **mandible** moving backward. **Whiplash** means double trauma for all the tissues, first by stretching and second by compression.

Even though I stated in the introduction that trauma would not be discussed, **whiplash** is such a common injury that it must be

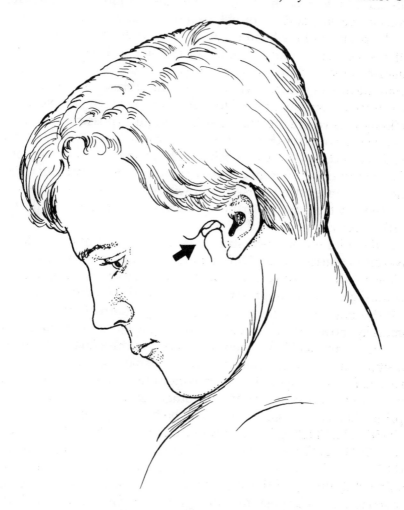

Figure 13. The forward flexion phase of whiplash. The arrow indicates force.

addressed. Anyone who has had a **whiplash** or neck injury is suspect for TMJ. Most of these people heal well and do not develop a problem. It takes a couple of minutes to check for problems in the TMJ, a couple minutes well spent. Now let us look at two more situations that commonly alter normal functioning.

Poor dental care can alter the normal functioning of the area whether it be poor **hygiene**, inappropriate removal of teeth, or poorly fitting dentures. If the normal resting position of the jaw is altered significantly, the stage is set for the inflammation of tissues, **muscle spasms**, and abnormal wear of the **disc**.

The position of the head on the neck, and the neck on the body, affects the position and function of the jaw. If the head becomes displaced forward, the amount of jaw opening becomes reduced. Examine this for yourself while you open and close your jaw in front of a mirror. Slouch your head forward and open your jaw. Now do a military tuck where the head is as far upright as possible, and open your jaw. About one-third of the opening is reduced with the head held in an extreme forward position. The change in tooth contact is also significantly different in the two positions. See if you can notice the subtle difference yourself. You will have more of an **overbite**, i.e. the top teeth move farther forward over the lower teeth, the farther forward your head is.

Early thinking in dentistry operated on the premise that an **overbite** contributed to TMJ symptoms. Some dentists may still follow this line of thinking. **Splints** designed to bring the lower jaw forward are still being prescribed to correct the **overbite.**

If the position of the head is restored to normal, the jaw will naturally move forward because most of the stresses on the tissue pulling it back will have been removed. By correcting faulty head position, and restoring normal resting position of the tongue, the jaw will find its proper place. **Repositioning** by means of a **splint** is not always necessary. There are other reasons why the use of **splints** may be necessary which will be discussed later.

THE BITE SHOULD NOT BE CHANGED THROUGH SPLINT-ING UNTIL THE HEAD IS ALIGNED PROPERLY ON THE NECK AND BODY. Proper alignment is present when the tip of the ear is in line with the tip of the shoulder as viewed from the side. Have someone view your posture to determine how far forward the tip of your ear is from the tip of your shoulder. Be sure you are not rounding your shoulder forward.

Medical
and
<u>Dental</u>
Considerations

edicine is an art as well as a science,
and the most important knowledge in medicine
to be learned and taught is the way the
human mind and body can summon innermost
resources to meet extraordinary challenges.
— Norman Cousins

Three

OVERVIEW

Chances are that if you begin to experience pain in your body you will go to your doctor. This is good because pain or illness tells you that something is wrong and a doctor who is a good diagnostician is solid gold. There are many dedicated competent doctors and dentists who administer the finest possible care for their patients. There are also poor diagnosticians who through bad judgement and egotism abuse their power. Practicing in the medical profession consciously, learning through each experience is humbling. And although great pride can be felt for a job well done, the best of us realizes that we are only an important player on a team. Look for humility.

So it is with great encouragement that I recommend if you have a TMJ problem or headaches, that you enter the health care system at this point, the doctor's or preferrably the dentist's office, but it is also with reservation. Controversy abounds in this area, and there is much diversity in thinking as to how to approach treatment of headaches and TMJ. This book will help equip you with knowledge so that you are better able to evaluate if you are being treated in the best way possible. We the practitioners are accountable to you. Hold us accountable.

Generally, practitioners do not like to be challenged. Personally, I like a patient who asks questions because it indicates to me that they are interested. A word of caution though when you challenge a plan of treatment. Do it with an open attitude in the spirit of inquiry. Most of us are doing the best we can with what we know.

The two main reasons why you should go to a doctor or dentist first, are that you need an overall coordinator of your care, and, there is a chance that something could be seriously wrong requiring medical attention. Almost all of the patients I treat have a **dysfunction** in one or more areas of their body. If it is amenable to the therapy I administer, the patient leaves improved. However, in a small percentage of cases a patient may not respond to treatment and further medical evaluation may be necessary to arrive at a different diagnosis. Or, there may be an underlying medical condition that requires some form of medical treatment to be administered and monitored, at the same time that a person is undergoing treatment for headaches or TMJ. When this is the case, a physician must be available to work with the radiologist, lab technicians, surgeons, etc. to interpret the data and orchestrate the case.

CHOOSING YOUR DOCTOR

You can look up physician in the yellow pages but you can't look up quarterback. And what you need is a good quarterback. You need someone to decide how and when the plays are going to get played. They do not do all the work. They coordinate the care. I have seen some great quarterbacking. When they are great they are great. But when they are not the results can be devastating. The management of a TMJ problem is complex. You need someone with competence and compassion. Do not compromise in this area.

You are not shopping for a VCR. You are screening someone to be your doctor. Before you choose your doctor, determine the things that are important to you and the things that are not that important. For example, it may not matter to you that your doctor is a particular sex. It may be very important to you that he/she listens to you or has a good bedside manner. Know what is important to you. Then begin to ask around, friends, neighbors, beauticians (great sources for all kinds of information), people in your exercise class. Word of mouth is the best advertisement. People know who the good practitioners are in a community. Then check them out for yourself. Someone who appealed to your racquetball partner may not appeal to you. This process takes time. Take the time.

Some suggested minimum requirements when screening for a doctor are the following. They should be a good diagnostician. You can base this on previous experience with this doctor or a recommendation from someone you trust. They should have a good background and training in TMJ. This is harder to assess since there is no uniform specialty certfication process. They should be a good listener. I have found that the patient almost always gives me the diagnosis if I listen carefully. And finally, out of respect for you as an individual, the doctor should have somewhat of a compassionate manner.

I believe you should make your decision intuitively. This is your body that you are going to entrust to this person. If there is a strained feeling between the two of you, or if there is something that you don't like about the practitioner, you probably will not be able to trust them. If you know beyond the shadow of a doubt your doctor is committed to you and your case, it is much easier to develop a trusting relationship. The bond between the doctor and the patient is a powerful force, instrumental in the healing process.

These principles hold true in searching for and choosing any practitioner that is going to be on your team. But they are most importantly applied when choosing your physician.

DENTAL CONSIDERATIONS

If a pain is experienced in the jaw, the first logical place to look is the teeth. A toothache from a common **cavity** could conceivably mimic any TMJ symptom, especially pain in the jaw. When a **cavity** begins to erode into the **pulp chamber** or **root canal** it can cause a great deal of local pain, as most of us can attest to, and also refer pain to another site. Dental origin should be suspected in every TMJ case.

Also, if the jaw bone becomes eroded, inflamed, or infected, pain can arise. This is referred to as **periodontal disease**. Inflammation of gum tissue around a tooth (**gingivitis**) left unattended, can affect the tooth and bone below. This is why good dental **hygiene**, regular check ups, cleaning of the teeth, and daily flossing, is so important. **Cavities** are not a main concern in the adult, since they tend to decrease in frequency the older we get. What is of concern is the maintenance of healthy gums, so that the teeth and their supporting bony structures (the jaw bone) do not deteriorate.

There are numerous other dental **pathologies** that can give rise to pain in the jaw but they are beyond the scope of this book. Your dentist is trained to evaluate for these. Clearing this area as a contributing cause of TMJ is imperative. Just a few of the common **pathologies** will now be presented.

Occasionally one of the bones of the jaw grows too large. When the **mandible** becomes larger in comparison to the upper jaw, the **mandible** is referred to as being **prognathic** and appears to protrude forward. When the **mandible** underdevelops and is too small in comparison to the upper jaw, the **mandible** is referred to as **retrognathic**, and appears to be positioned too far back. It is also possible that the bones on one side can become larger, causing asymmetry of the face. When any of these situations are present, the method of choice to correct the problem is surgery. Surgery to correct bony abnormalities is referred to as **orthognathic surgery**.

The other function the dentist plays is determining if your teeth are giving proper support to the jaw joint. If there is inadequate posterior support from the teeth due to their absence or if the teeth are asymmetrical, the bite will be imbalanced. And here is where the controversy begins. There seem to be two main camps that dentists fall into. The first camp believes that it is important to make the bite more symmetrical through utilizing **splints**, filing down or building up teeth. The second camp believes the muscular system through **occlusal** overstressing such as clenching and grinding contributes to the problem and treats the problem behaviorally. How your case is handled will be determined by which camp your dentist belongs to. Perhaps in no other area have so many worked so long and hard to arrive at such controversy. And yet it is the dentists who have pioneered in this area. Most dentists now subscribe to a muscle based theory rather than an **occlusion** based theory as to the cause of TMJ. But not everyone agrees as to how it is best treated. The use of **splints** in the management of TMJ is likely to remain a controversial topic.

The **occlusion** helps determine the position of the jaw along with tongue position, the position of the neck, and the muscles of the head and neck. Gross inadequacies in quality and quantity of support from the teeth may need to be corrected. This according to some dentists requires the use of a **splint** sometimes referred to as an interocclusal appliance. **Splints** are usually made of a hard acrylic resin and can be worn on the lower or upper teeth. **Splints** serve three primary purposes. They are used to improve the mechanics of the joint, improve the function of the muscles by restoring the normal resting length of muscle and reducing spasm, and protect the teeth from excessive loading as in the case of clenching and grinding.

Splints are usually worn all of the time at the beginning of the therapy. Some are taken out in the day and only worn at night. People who clench and/or grind at night (**bruxism**) often find relief from a night **splint** or a night guard which can be soft or hard. Even if clenching is not controlled with the **splint** the teeth will be protected from wearing. These have individual success rates for control of clenching behavior. It is up to your dentist and therapist to determine if an appliance is indicated and how it should be worn.

Splints fall into two basic categories. One type of **splint** is designed to disengage the **occlusion**, thereby restoring vertical dimension. Vertical dimension is the distance between the top and bottom teeth. Increasing this distance, is thought to restore normal resting length to the muscles of the jaw, and improve the mechanics of the joint. **Splints** place a gentle downward pull on the jaw, which disengages the **condyle** of the **mandible** from its deeply seated position in the **fossa** of the **temporal bone**, thereby relieving pressure on the joint structures. This is referred to as a **resting splint**, which simply rests the jaw. The second type of **splint** is designed to reposition the **mandible** either forward or to one side so that the **condyle's** position on the **disc** is improved.

A **resting splint** is less invasive than a **repositioning splint** in that when it is time to come out of the **splint**, it is simply worn for a decreasing number of hours per day. When the jaw is repositioned forward or to the side often it must then be permanently fixed in that position. This requires **bracing, bonding,** and/or various other procedures which will be discussed next.

Procedures which permanently alter the **occlusion** are usually performed by an **orthodontist. Orthodontics** is the art and science of correcting the position of the teeth, through the use of gradual constant mechanical pressure. The use of **braces** is the most common method used in **orthodontics**. Techniques of **bracing** have been so refined that now the materials can be made transparent and with far less wiring. Also, it is possible to have some types of **braces** attach to the inside of the teeth. And while it is not easy to learn to talk with the intrusion of the **bracing** material in the mouth, it is certainly more cosmetically pleasing.

The role that the **orthodontist** plays is that of assuring an effective and stable **occlusion**. They do this in a variety of ways. The most common way, as mentioned above, is by the use of **braces**. The use of these fixed appliances can move teeth to a new position, raise or lower teeth, and widen or narrow the arches of the mouth. Other procedures which can balance or even an **occlusion** are **capping**, if a tooth is deteriorating, or **bonding**, if a tooth needs to be built up. Also, teeth can be filed down if they are too high.

The purpose of all of these procedures is to equilibrate the bite to achieve the most desirable relationship between the top and bottom teeth. These methods should only be utilized when satisfactory elimination of symptoms has been accomplished. THESE PROCEDURES ARE IRREVERSIBLE AND SHOULD BE PRESCRIBED AND ADMINISTERED WITH GREAT CAUTION! Further, it should be noted that all of these procedures are costly and sometimes require years of committment to the process in order to effect change. Nevertheless, when conservative management has failed, it may be necessary to apply these techniques. Second opinions are a good idea.

If a **repositioning splint** has been used to stabilize the jaw, and the desired result has been obtained, one of two options is available, depending on the specifics of each case. In option one, the patient is slowly weaned off the **splint**, and/or adjustments may be made on the **splint** which allows the jaw to return to its original position before treatment began. In cases where the **disc** has been 'recaptured" or healed this works quite nicely. However, sometimes it may be necessary to permanently move the teeth into a position that matches the position that the jaw is in, while in the **splint**. For example, if symptoms such as clicking, pain, and deviation to the side are present upon removal of the **splint**, and, these symptoms are controlled with the **splint**, permanently altering the bite in order to stabilize the jaw may be indicated.

Look for a dentist who works conservatively first. Approximately 80-90% of all TMJ patients are of the **MPD** or muscle type who can get by with a **resting splint** or no **splint** at all. In these cases physical therapy and behavioral techniques such as **biofeedback** are what is indicated. Among my colleagues, the general consensus is that we prefer to work with patients initially without **splints** if they fall into the **MPD** category.

On occasion, insertion of a **splint** gives dramatic reduction of all or a significant part of the pain. In the early 1960's, long before TMJ was popular, my mother had a **splint** made that she reports greatly decreased the pain down her leg. We do not fully understand why the position of the **mandible** affects other parts of the body in some people but we have observed that it does. The rule is to do **noninvasive therapy** first, then move on to other procedures if necessary. Another rule, GET THE RIGHT SPLINT!

The second logical place to look after the teeth have been cleared is the head and neck area itself. The medical **pathologies** that are possible here are as varied as the dental ones. A good diagnostician will do what is referred to as a systems review which reviews all of the major systems of the body to get a clue as to whether an **organic disease** process might be going on in the body. X-rays in various forms may need to be taken. If there is no suspicion for **disease** you may be referred for treatment pending further evaluation if treatment is not successful. But again, in a small number of cases pain in this area can arise from more serious pathology such as tumor or systemic illness and you may need to be evaluated for these conditions.

MEDICAL CONSIDERATIONS

Have you ever stopped to consider that when you go to the doctor with a complaint that the cause could literally be anything. That doctor has to be a detective, a sleuth, Angela Lansbury herself. It could be something serious, something minor, or even everyday stress. Perhaps because diagnosis is so complex the physician often blames the patient's psyche. However, it is the physician's reponsibility to synthesize all of the medical and behavioral factors that are contributing to the patient's pain. Often, all that is necessary is a good solid referral to a practitioner who can help in the treatment of the problem.

From the medical history, presenting symptoms, clinical exam and laboratory data, the physician can determine if the problem is one of **organic disease** or **dysfunction**. Barring serious **pathology**, the patient falls into one of two categories, that of a primary joint problem which consist of 10-20% of the cases, or that of a primary muscle problem, **MPD**, which consists of 80-90% of the cases. And even this may be a conservative estimate. The latest research suggests that perhaps only 7-10% of all cases are true mechanical problems of the joint. That means that perhaps as many as 93% of all TMJ cases may be **MPD** related. This book deals primarily with the management of **MPD** cases.

It should be noted that these are general categories. If someone has a primary joint problem, a large part of the pain could be muscular in origin. Similarly, a person with a primary muscular problem can, through **muscle spasm**, develop a significant mechanical problem. As treatment progresses one develops more insight as to the actual cause of the pain. The categories of mechanical and muscular are useful but are not absolute.

Medical management as it relates to **MPD** cases is outlined in illustrious detail in a book written by Dr. Janet Travell called Myofascial Pain and Dysfunction. Her work has contributed much to the body of knowledge concerning muscle. There are a number of perpetuating factors, which if not corrected, maintain the pain and spasm cycle. The following is a shortened version of the management of these factors.

A simple example will illustrate the importance of identifying perpetuating factors. If you slip on a banana peel and hurt your back, it would be a good idea to pick up the banana peel and throw it out so that you do not slip on it again. Muscles are sensitive to a variety of stimuli and they respond to stimuli in two ways: by developing **trigger points**, which are areas of sensitivity within the muscle, and by going into spasm. Removing the stimuli which can irritate muscle removes the perpetuating factors or the banana peel so that treatment can be more effective.

The first area that contributes to perpetuating the pain and spasm cycle is the psyche. Our attitudes about our lives can influence how much pain we experience. Anxiety and depression tend to increase the level of pain we experience. On days when you just don't feel well sometimes it is hard to determine if you actually have more pain, or if you just don't feel well. In a later section of this book we will explore the many ways in which your mind contributes to how you perceive your pain.

Mechanical stresses can lead to strain of the muscles by making them work harder than they need to. Common stresses are poor posture, leg length discrepancies, constriction of clothing, poorly designed furniture, and shoulder bags carried on the same side of the body. These factors will be presented in considerable detail in a later section of this book.

Vitamin and mineral deficiencies, particularly lack of B1, B6, B12, C, Folic Acid, Calcium, Iron, and Potassium, increase the irritability of the **Central Nervous System** and muscle. When these important substances are not present, the metabolism of the body as it relates to muscle contraction, gets interferred with. Vitamin supplements should be recommended and your progress monitored by your doctor. It is a part of the overall treatment plan, not the entire plan. Beware of practitioners who sell and promote extensive lines of vitamins out of their office. Nevertheless, it is an important aspect.

Hypothyroidism and **hypoglycemia** interfere with the energy metabolism of the body. Decreased function of the thyroid and decreased blood sugar levels give rise to irritability of muscle. Again, these factors are to be weighed and monitored by your doctor.

A chronic infection can be a complicating factor in why the pre-scribed therapy is not progressing. A common cold sore, which is the herpes simplex virus, sinusitis, or a chronic urinary tract infec-tion are all examples of a chronic low grade infection. A universal experience is the achiness accompanied by the flu. If you have had a previous injury, you may find that you have more pain in an area of the body that was injured, when you have the flu.

A particular complicating factor with TMJ is allergies. The epi-sodic sneezing, full, and often blocked nasal passages, itchiness in the throat, and tearing puts stress on the entire head and neck complex. The presence of allergies can predispose a person to develop an upper respiratory infection, a common perpetuating factor for TMJ and headaches.

Disrupted sleep patterns can increase irritability of muscle and lead to increased pain. This pain can then further disrupt sleep. Often after the first few therapy sessions my patients comment that they are sleeping deeper and longer. It is often the first sign of improvement. When the person's normal sleep patterns are re-stored, particularly long deep sleep, the body can begin to get the rest that it needs to replenish itself and heal.

All of these aspects may not need to be addressed in your case. Just be aware of them as complicating factors. If your therapy is not going according to plan, it may be that one of these factors is operating.

An important role that the physician or dentist has in the medical management of headaches and TMJ is prescribing medication. The judicious use of the various drugs available can do much to break the pain and spasm cycle, as well as enhance the effects of therapy. And while there is potential for abuse in this area, I view the short term use of medication as assisting in the promotion of the desired **physiological** changes.

There are a few categories of drugs that are commonly prescribed for headache and TMJ. **Analgesics** and **anti-inflammatory** medications relieve both inflammation and pain. There are a variety on the market. If you are going to Mt. Everest, best take Bayer to be safe. But for the rest of us, I'd say find the ones that work the best for you and stick with it, whether that be Tylenol or Aspirin. These two are both considered analgesics, i.e. painkillers. Ibuprofen, which is sold as Nuprin, Medipren, and Advil, and probably a few more by now, is considered to be primarily an **anti-inflammatory** medication. This is becoming a very popular choice.

Another commonly prescribed medication is that of **muscle relaxants**. In addition to reducing **muscle spasm,** some reduce anxiety, which helps decrease the psychological stress which accompanies pain. .These can be very effective in reducing **muscle spasm**. However, since many of them are habit forming, short term therapy is recommended for their use, i.e. 4-6 weeks.

The next category of drugs often prescribed for headache and TMJ is the **antidepressants**. They are administered in doses much lower than ones used in treating depression. Elavil, or amitriptyline, is the most common of the **antidepressants** prescribed to control pain. This is often prescribed to help restore normal sleep patterns. In some cases this can be very helpful. There is one other category of drug which is being used quite effectively in the control of headache. These medications are referred to as **beta blockers** and they work by blocking pain signals at certain synapses or junctions between nerves. A **beta blocker** often prescribed is Inderal.

Medication has its greatest effect three days after you begin to take it. This delay occurs because it takes the body several days to build a high enough blood concentration level for it to be therapeutically effective. It is important to take medication regularly and in the prescribed dosage, in order to maintain this high concentration level. Medication needs to be taken for a period of at least 4 weeks to receive the maximum benefit. It should go without saying that patients need to be monitored closely by their dentists or physicians when they are on medication. The purpose of this supervision is to make note of the therapeutic effects as well as check for side effects. Further, regulation of the dosage may be in order.

SURGICAL CONSIDERATIONS

Occasionally surgery is indicated for the correction of a TMJ problem. If the **disc** is found to be improperly positioned, it may need to be repositioned surgically. If the **disc** is torn, frayed or has deteriorated, it may need to be removed or replaced.

A **silastic disc** implant can be inserted in place of the body's natural **disc**. This is mostly necessary in cases of trauma. The **silastic** implant is attached to the surrounding joint tissue. Where there is inadequate tissue to attach the implant to, due to trauma or deterioration, the **disc** is simply removed.

This procedure, called **menisectomy**, is quite commonly done in the knee. Surgeons have come to appreciate that saving as much of the natural **disc** as possible is preferable. But when it is necessary to remove it, these patients seem to do quite well.

If the joint surfaces are badly worn, a jaw joint implant may be indicated. As bone begins to break down, the lower jaw can begin to shrink in relation to the upper jaw, giving the face an unbalanced look. Both the ball and socket parts of the joint are replaced, which restores normal functioning to the area. A good cosmetic result can be obtained with this surgery. Although this type of surgery is not as common as it is for the hip and knee joints, it is gaining in popularity. Only a small percentage of patients are considered candidates for this surgery.

If surgery is indicated in your case, here is what you can generally expect. Surgery is done under general anesthesia as an inpatient. You will need to spend a few days in the hosptial recuperating, at which time you will be eating soft foods until the area heals. Normal functioning of the TMJ usually returns within 4-6 weeks. You will most likely be referred to physical therapy to help prevent adhesions from forming, to promote healing, and to restore normal range of motion as quickly as possible. Cosmetically, only a small scar in front of the ear remains, which is covered by the hair.

When cases are diagnosed properly, and the surgery is successful, recovery is usually full and complete. Following any surgery, complications are possible such as infection or the loss of nerve supply, in this case to the face. But generally this is a relatively common procedure and a good result can be expected. Of course a good surgeon helps!

The newest medical breakthrough in the area of TMJ is **arthroscopic surgery**. This technique gives the surgeon the ability to view the inside of the joint and perform simple procedures through a scope which is inserted into the joint by puncturing the skin and soft tissues. The scope is attached to a television monitor, which allows for viewing of the structures. It requires great skill on the part of the surgeon since the screen is two dimensional and the joint is three dimensional.

The **arthroscope** makes possible visualization of the joint and most of its structures in great detail. It can identify torn and/or displaced **discs**, degenerative changes, and the presence of scar tissue and inflammation within the joint. Miniature surgical instruments can be inserted through the scope and certain procedures can be performed such as removal of scar tissue and adhesions.

Although the introduction of this technique is a real breakthrough in the medical management of TMJ, there are some limitations. Not all areas of the joint can be reached with the scope, and the types of procedures that can be performed through the scope are limited, due to its small size. For example, a **disc** would not be able to be replaced using the **arthroscopic** method.

The complications that arise as a result of **arthroscopic surgery** are considerably less than those of the open-joint method. However, the possibility remains for infection, loss of function of the nerves to the face, as well as risks associated with anesthesia. And there is a one complication which is unique to this type of surgery. A slight chance exists that the tip of the scope or one of the instruments could break off inside the joint. If this happens the surgeon would move directly to an open-joint method to remedy the situation.

The TMJ is a relatively difficult area to reach surgically since it is deeply embedded in the tissues of the face. As the arthroscopic technique becomes more readily available, it will be of enormous benefit in reducing the risks of surgery, as well as significantly decrease recovery time. If it has been determined that you require surgery, you may want to inquire as to whether someone in your area is performing surgery on the TMJ through the **arthroscope**. You may be a candidate for this procedure.

RADIOGRAPHIC EXAMINATION

The discovery of X-rays in 1895 revolutionized medical and surgical diagnosis. Prior to that time diagnosis was determined by clinical exam and laboratory data alone. A **radiograph** makes it possible to view anatomical structures that were previously unobservable. Diagnosis can now be made easier and with greater accuracy through the use of **radiographs**.

Various forms of imaging are used to detect abnormalities in structure and function, identify stages of disease, give information to guide the **splint** therapy, and help solve treatment failures. Images provide details of the bony anatomy, such as the surface contours of bone, which should be smooth, round and regular, i.e. no "break" in the image which would signify fracture. Images also show the position of the bones in relation to each other, position of the **disc**, and the functioning of the joint.

There are four types of films commonly used in evaluating the TMJ. They are **plain films** (transcranial radiographs), **tomograms** (**CT scans**), **arthrograms**, and the most recent addition **magnetic resonance imaging (MRI)**. These will now be discussed and an example of each will be included so that you can see the similarities as well as the differences between the images.

A **plain film** or transcranial radiograph, as in all films, is a negative. Just as you must hold the negatives from your camera up to the light to view them, X-rays are viewed on a light viewing box. Denser tissues appear whiter on X-ray so the bone will be the most prominent structure visible. Any information on the soft tissues such as the **ligaments** or **disc** can only be inferred from the position of the bones because they are only somewhat visible. The strength of the **plain film** is that it can be done inexpensively in the dentist's office with minimal radiation exposure. It gives valuable information on the quality and position of the bones. You can tell very little about the **disc** or the function of the joint from an X-ray, but it is an excellent screening device and a good place to start the evaluation. See Figure 1. Note that in Figures 1, 4, 5, and 6 you will see a term used called **articular eminence**. This is the most anterior portion of the **temporal bone**. The **condyle** of the **mandible** comes in contact with this eminence when the jaw is fully opened.

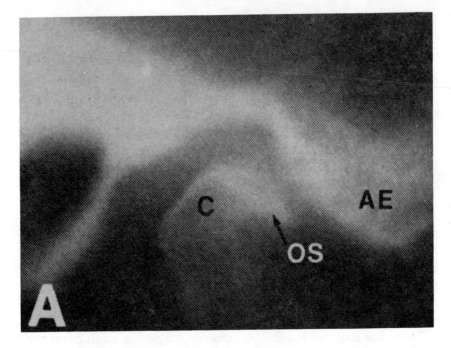

Figure 1. Plain film of the TMJ showing degenerative joint disease. A well defined bone spur (OS) is present on the anterior surface of the condyle. The condyle of the madible is labeled "C", and the surface on which the condyle glides is labeled "AE" for articular eminence.

Reproduced by permission from, Blaschke, Donald P., and Bergeron, R. Thomas.: The temporomandibular joint. In Bergeron, R. Thomas, Osborn, Anne G., and Som, Peter M., editors: Head and Neck Imaging Excluding the Brain, St. Louis, 1984, The C. V. Mosby Co.

A **tomogram** combines the use of radiation physics, electronics and computer science to produce imaginative imagery. It adds a degree of accuracy over a **plain film**. An X-ray tries to capture a three dimensional structure on a two dimensional film which cannot be an accurate representation of an area. That is why at least two views and often four views of the same area have to be taken, to improve accuracy.

A **tomogram** is an image of a slice of tissue taken at a particular depth. This allows for a clearer differentiation of structure and enables us to detect problems that were not as clearly seen on **plain film**. During the procedure, the area to be scanned passes into the

CT "tube". Images are taken and then computed. Figure 2 depicts how slices of tissue are viewed.

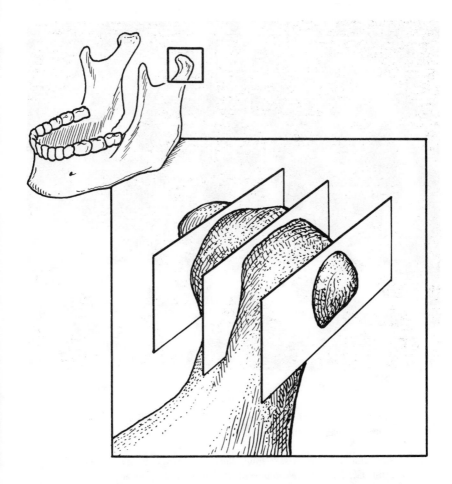

Figure 2. This illustrates how slices or sections of the TMJ can be viewed by tomography. Lateral, central, or medial portions of the condyle can be computed.

The bony anatomy can be seen very well, and **disc** position can be detected from a **tomographic** image. The disadvantages of **CT scanning** are that it is expensive, and it must be done at a center which has a scanner. When indicated, it is a powerful tool, which gives quite accurate information. Figures 3 and 4 show examples of two types of **CT scans**.

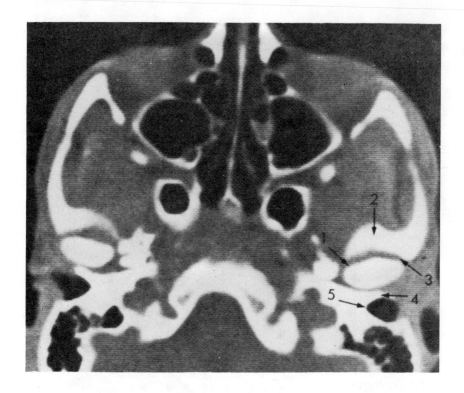

Figure 3. Computed tomography of the TMJ. 1. condyle, 2. fossa of temporal bone, 3. joint space, 4. temporal bone, 5. ear

Reproduced by permission from, Blaschke, Donald P., and Osborn, Anne G.: The mandible and teeth. In Bergeron, R. Thomas, Osborn, Anne G., and Som, Peter M., editors: Head and Neck Imaging Excluding the Brain, St. Louis, 1984, The C. V. Mosby Co.

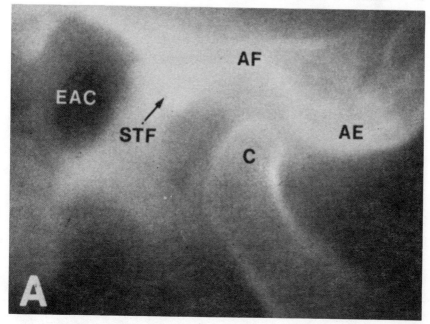

Figure 4. Computed tomography of the TMJ. "C" is the condyle, "AF" is the articular fossa, "AE" is the articular eminence, "EAC" is the ear.

Reproduced by permission from, Blaschke, Donald P., and Bergeron, R. Thomas.: The temporomandibular joint. In Bergeron, R. Thomas, Osborn, Anne G., and Som, Peter M., editors: Head and Neck Imaging Excluding the Brain, St. Louis, 1984, The C. V. Mosby Co.

An **arthrogram** is the most common diagnostic procedure used to rule out a mechanical joint problem, which includes approximately 10-20% of all TMJ cases. An anesthetic is administered to the area so that discomfort is minimized. A contrast medium (something that will show up on X-ray) is introduced to the joint, and a film is taken of the area. In an **arthrogram** what you observe is the contrast material, and you infer the position, size, and shape of the **disc**. The contrast medium is sometimes removed after the procedure. **Tomograms** are usually taken at the same time, with the mouth in various positions of opening. Often the image of the joint can be observed on a fluorescent screen and videotaped, which is called **flouroscopy**. This produces a picture of the inside of the joint during movement. This is referred to as a dynamic radiograph because it gives a moving picture of the joint. Dynamic radiographs are extremely helpful because they identify where in the range of motion the problem occurs.

No other technique gives the amount of information about the **disc** than the **arthrogram**, which is why its use is so widespread. Although it is somewhat more invasive, in that injections are required and radiation exposure is higher than a **radiograph**, it remains the standard procedure for diagnosis of a mechanical problem in the TMJ. See Figure 5.

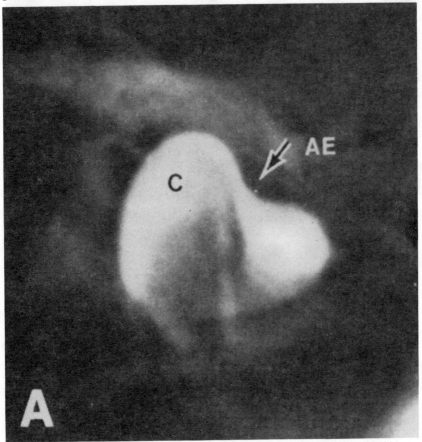

Figure 5. Abnormal TMJ arthrogram. The lower joint space is seen as the white area. The arrow depicts an area which is seen as a convexity at the joint space. This illustrates an abnormality in the relationship between the surface of the disc, the joint space, and the condyle. "C" is the condyle. "AE is the articular eminence of the temporal bone.

Reproduced by permission from, Blaschke, Donald P., and Bergeron, R. Thomas.: The temporomandibular joint. In Bergeron, R. Thomas, Osborn, Anne G., and Som, Peter M., editors: Head and Neck Imaging Excluding the Brain, St. Louis, 1984, The C. V. Mosby Co.

The **arthrogram** determines if the **disc** is "reducable', i.e. able to be repositioned, using an appliance, or if it must be surgically repositioned. It will also determine if the **disc** is torn or needs replacement. The diagnostic term used to describe a mechanical problem in the joint is **internal derangement (ID)**. So the **arthrogram** will help determine what kind of **ID** you have.

Usually the **disc** slips forward (anterior displacement) so that when the jaw opens, the **disc**, which is already forward, will not allow further motion of the **mandible**. Jaw opening is limited in this case, and this situation is referred to as a close locked problem. The amount of forward displacement of the **disc** determines whether the problem can be corrected clinically, by the use of a **repositioning splint**, or if surgery is necessary.

Another situation can occur where the **condyle** can jump over an area of the **disc**, at which point there may be a click or pop. These problems can often be managed clinically. But in the case of limited opening due to a forward slipped **disc** these may or may not be clinically manageable.

My patients report to me that they go into the **arthrogram** expecting the worst, but that they actually were not as uncomfortable as they thought they were going to be. A few have some soreness in the joint for several days. Occasionally their symptoms may increase for a short time. What has also been reported is a decrease in the pain. This may be explained by the fact that pressure may be relieved during the procedure.

In summary, visualization of the soft tissues of the TMJ as well as **disc** position, size, and shape are possible through the use of an **arthrogram**. Along with **tomograms** of the TMJ, an accurate diagnosis can be made as to the integrity of the joint in general and specifically the **disc**.

The state of the art in imaging is **magnetic resonance imaging (MRI)**. It has the potential to replace **CT scans** and **arthrography** in TMJ diagnosis. Briefly, and very simply, here is how **MRI** works. Through the use of a surface coil, a body coil, and a very large superconductive magnet, an electromagnetic field is created around the body, which aligns the hydrogen protons of the tissues. The alignment of the protons in the field can be plotted out as data points, which can then be computed to form an image. An example of an **MRI** is given in Figure 6.

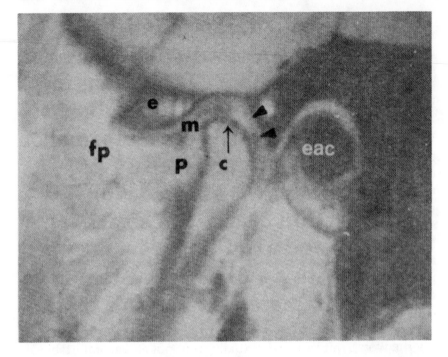

Figure 6. Magnetic Resonance Image of the TMJ. "c" is the condyle, "m" is the disc, "p" is the lateral pterygoid muscle, "fp" is the fat pad, "e" is the articular eminence of the temporal bone, and "eac" is the ear.

Reproduced by permission from "Normal and Abnormal TMJ: MR Imaging with Surface Coil," by Dr. Richard Katzberg, et al, Radiology 158:pgs 183-189, January 1986.

The use of a technique which utilizes electromagnetic energy to obtain images instead of radiation is a real breakthrough. This imaging technique is safer for the patient and gives clearer images than any other film, as can be seen in Figure 6. The disadvantage is that, like **CT scanning**, it is expensive. But stay tuned. This area shows great promise in becoming the standard for practice in the not too distant future.

IN SUMMARY

An X-ray gives a picture of the bony aspects of the joint. A **tomogram (CT scan)** does it better, but not as good as a **MRI**, and you get the soft tissues too. **Arthrograms** give you dynamic information but are the most invasive. If you are in the 10-20% group who has a mechanical joint problem you will probably have an arthrogram since **CT scans** and **MRI** are expensive, $600 a shot (literally).

A word of caution about imaging. They are not 100% accurate. There are such occurrences as false positives and false negatives. This means that what you see is not always what is there. And diagnoses may be made incorrectly because the angle or positioning may not be quite right to view the problem. As the quality of the image improves, so does the accuracy. However, the final diagnosis should be based on the combined evidence from clinical examination, other laboratory data, and X-ray. The X-ray report should merely verify what you suspected clinically in most cases.

At least 80% of all TMJ cases, and a large majority of headache cases are **myofascial** in origin. Yet there are no imaging techniques to evaluate muscle. Spasm, tightness, and weakness remain clinical phenomenon that we can see and feel but have a more difficult time measuring. Everyone agrees that muscle tightness and spasm often cause pain and yet it is one of the most difficult areas in which to obtain objective measurements.

HEADACHES

Volumes have been written on the subject of headaches and yet an estimated 45 million people continue to suffer from the chronic pain of headache. It appears as if the common cold and headache are two afflictions medicine has not been able to remedy. Many people have been helped with various forms of therapy, but it seems as if we cannot get a grasp on the underlying mechanisms causing headache. Some new thoughts on the subject are that the different types of headaches are perhaps not so different after all. Research is presently being aimed at looking at common factors which may contribute to the cause of all types of headaches.

Headaches are not life threatening, and yet anyone who has had one can attest to how bad you can feel. A Harris Poll showed that in

1986 businesses lost $55 million in absenteeism and health care costs due to headaches. The National Center for Health Statistics estimated that children lost 1.3 million days of school due to headaches. Further, we as a nation have come to rely on drugs as the main form of treatment. One evening while watching television I counted ten commercials for analgesics. Drugs only treat the symptom, not the cause of the headache.

At least 80% of headaches are muscular in origin. There are often triggering mechanisms such as allergies, viruses, and dietary influences, but muscle appears to play a great role in headache production. That is probably why programs which utilize treatments such as biofeedback and relaxation techniques report an 85-90% success rate. In a large number of these cases, physical therapy can also provide a dramatic reduction in headaches.

So it would appear that one of the underlying causes of a large percentage of headaches is muscle. And we know how to treat muscle effectively. By restoring proper length through stretching, promoting relaxation through massage and other modalities, and restoring strength through graded exercise we can get much closer to the cause than by masking the problem with an analgesic.

Many different types of headaches have been identified but most of them fall into three basic categories: migraine, cluster, and tension. These constitute 95% of all headaches. The other 5% are related to disease states such as tumors or systemic illness which this book does not address.

In the classic migraine the headache is often preceeded by what is called an aura where spots or lights appear or a particular feeling is present. A throbbing unilateral pain is common. It occurs more often in women and commonly around or during menstruation. Nausea and vomiting, as well as light and noise sensitivity, can accompany these headaches. They can last several days. Many of my patients tell me that they stay in bed until they pass.

Cluster headaches are the most excruciating, lasting from minutes to hours, coming on suddenly as a stabbing pain near the eye, causing tearing and a blocked or runny nose. The pain is sometimes so severe that people have been known to commit bizarre acts in the midst of one of these. They come in clusters, sometimes several in a day lasting for weeks or months then disappear only to reappear at a later date. Cluster headaches occur more often in men. One common characteristic is that the people who tend to get them have a ruddy leathery weathered look to their faces.

Tension headaches are generalized and dull, affecting the entire head. Some people report a viselike grip around the head. They last for varying amounts of time and are by far the most common type of headache.

Other types of headaches have been identified such as vascular, sinus, hunger, and hangover. Some people report an increase in their headache during sex particularly at orgasm. Others experience an ease in the pain after sex. These other types are subdivisions of the three main categories. There is considerable overlap and commonality to them all.

A symptom which often accompanies TMJ is headache. Two patterns are the most prevalent, both of which belong in the tension category. The first is one in which the pain begins in the muscles at the base of the skull and radiates up over the back of the head into the forehead. The second begins over the jaw joints usually on one side and ends in the temples or top of the head. Other common ones are a visegrip around the head, and ones that begin in the forehead. Migraines are sometimes present.

For more specific information on the subject of headaches, I will refer you to an excellent book called, Headaches Aren't Forever, written by Dr. Gerald Smith. Dr. Smith is one of the leading dental experts in this country on TMJ and headaches. His book is listed in the bibliography.

The muscular system gives the most amount of sensory information to the **Central Nervous System** than any other system of the body. The nervous system functions in large part based on the the kind of information it is receiving from the muscles. The muscular system must be free from restriction so that it can give proper sensory information to the **Central Nervous System**. The next section of this book discusses how to restore the natural balance to the musculoskeletal system so that the stresses to the body can be minimized.

FINAL NOTE

ONCE THE PHYSICIAN HAS RULED OUT DISEASE HE/SHE SHOULD REFER YOU TO OTHER PROFESSIONALS WHO ARE TRAINED TO TREAT HEADACHES AND THE TMJ. My preference of course is a physical therapist.

Physical

Therapy

Management

e should believe only in deeds;
words go for nothing everywhere.
— Fernando Rojas

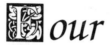
Four

OVERVIEW

Life is movement!

Many movements occur in our bodies without our even knowing it, such as the **diaphragm** rising and falling and the heart pumping rhythmically. Many of us who enjoy "people watching" are observing not only how people dress and present themselves to the world but also how they move. My cat thinks that the Tender Vittles flying across the kitchen ɹoor by a swat from his paw are much more interesting than the ones sitting in his dish. As a child I remember going to the Museum of Science and Industry in Chicago and being fascinated by the displays on various movements in the universe in the Hall of Motion. We human beings move about in interesting and unique ways, and are intrigued by things that move. Movement is an integral part of life.

The bones that form the skeleton and the muscles of the body are the supporting structure for the movement system. The **Central Nervous System (CNS)** through its millions of nerves and its complex interconnecting network drives the system. By moving in habitual ways, straining to perform tasks, withstanding falls and accidents, developing tightness and weakness in muscles due to the effects of gravity and inactivity, and developing poor postural habits, this system undergoes enormous amounts of strain. It is a resilient system absorbing and dissipating shock and **phys-**

iologically adapting to the loads or stresses we place upon it. But once the **physiological** adaptive capacity is exhausted something in the system has to give and that is often when we experience pain. When we have pain we change the way in which we move, sometimes limiting the amount of movement. Since movement is vital in maintaining the normal physiology or functioning of the body, this further strains the musculoskeletal system.

So a major goal of treatment of the TMJ is to restore normal movement of the jaw. But many aspects of treatment must be addressed before that goal can be reached. These will be discussed in the various sections of this chapter.

The first aspect of treatment is the promotion of healing by reducing pain and **muscle spasm**. The second aspect of treatment is the restoration of normal range of motion in both quality and quantity, to the jaw, neck, shoulder, and any other joint of the body that may be contributing to the pain. This includes restoring motion to a system called the **craniosacral** system which includes the **sutures** (joints) of the **cranium** (head).

The third aspect of treatment is the improvement of the overall posture of the body and specifically the forward head posture. The fourth aspect of treatment includes restoring normal **physiological** functioning to the head and neck areas. This is accomplished through establishing normal tongue position, improving the breathing pattern, improving swallowing, and through various body awareness exercises. The fifth aspect of treatment is education in proper body mechanics to minimize reoccurence of the problem. Since muscle is considered to be a prime factor in contributing to TMJ this is where our discussion will begin.

MUSCLE

There are approximately 696 muscles in the body, depending on how you count them. At a weight of 150 pounds at least sixty pounds of your body weight is muscle. Muscle is the single largest component of the body and yet is the most neglected structure to be considered in medical diagnosis. In many medical schools dissection of the musculoskeletal system is low priority. Many medical students do not even dissect this system. And yet one of the most common complaints a general practitioner will hear from his or her patient will arise from a problem with a musculoskeletal structure.

Muscle is highly innervated with nerve tissue and rich in blood supply which makes it an extremely sensitive structure. It receives an enormous amount of sensory information from the **CNS** and supplies equally as much information back into the **CNS**. The muscle, through its enormous blood flow, is sensitive to the body's metabolism and also affects the overall metabolism through the creation of energy. In Chapter 2 we discussed how low blood sugar and low thyroid function increased irritability of muscle. Some of us will recall from BIOLOGY 101 the process that eluded most of us at the time called the **Kreb Cycle** which actually creates the fuel we need for the body to function. That process occurs in the muscle. Muscle is a vital system of the body contributing greatly to overall functioning of the organism. Due to the powerful influence of this system, many of the improvements gained when muscle is treated and restored to normal go way beyond just pain control. When muscle function improves, the entire **physiology** of the body is affected for the better.

Muscle can respond to the various stresses we place upon it in a variety of ways. It can contract, thereby supplying us with the "muscle" to complete a task, and when the task is complete, it can relax. Contraction and relaxation are the two things that muscles do. When a muscle fails to relax, it may stay in a contracted state and we call that a **muscle spasm**. Most of us have experienced a charlie horse in our calf. **Muscle spasms** can be quite painful. They usually pass with time, a long soak in the tub, or by massaging it out.

But when an area undergoes prolonged strain or when a person holds tension in an area such as clenching the jaw, the muscles respond by maintaining prolonged muscle contractions, developing taut bands, and developing areas within the muscle which become extremely sensitive. These hyperirritable focuses in muscle are called **trigger points (t.p.'s)**. See Figure 1.

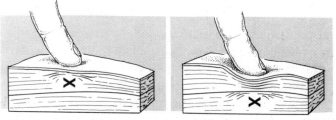

Figure 1. Schematic drawing of trigger points in various layers of muscle. As you move across the muscle belly the palpation finger rolls over this area, which makes it easily identifiable. Often t.p.'s are found in tight bands of muscle fibers.

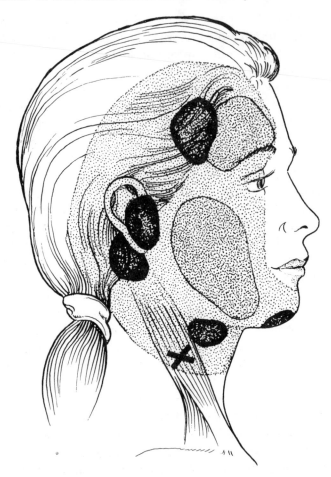

Figure 2. The trigger area marked X in the sternocleidomastoid (SCLM) muscle of the neck was stimulated and the distribution of pain referral was plotted. Darker areas represent greater focuses of pain. Pain is experienced at sites <u>distant</u> from the source. It is possible that pain in the TMJ could be caused by a trigger point in the SCLM muscle.

Trigger points can cause pain locally or can refer pain to another area. They may be the primary cause of TMJ, or may be part of the cause of the overall pain. They are a common cause of headache. **Trigger points** can become sensitive in response to a joint becoming tight. Figure 2 is an example of a referred pain to the head from a **t.p.** in the neck. As you can see the pain is experienced in the head, ear, jaw and chin as a result of stimulation of the point in the neck muscle. What this means is that the problem is actually in the neck muscle, but the person <u>perceives</u> it to be in the head and face.

Now let's locate a **trigger point** in one of your muscles. Take your middle finger and place it on your cheek in the belly of the **masseter muscle**. See if you can find an area that is more sensitive than the rest of the muscle. You may also feel a taut band in the muscle especially if you clench your teeth habitually.

The presence of a **t.p.** in an area strongly suggests that the area is being strained. Their presence should not be overlooked in the overall treatment plan. All **t.p.**'s in the head, neck, and shoulder need to be desensitized through treatment. This is especially true of ones which when stimulated, intensify the pain that the patient complains of. For example, if while pressing on a **t.p.** in the neck the patient reports the start of a headache they often experience, that point must be desensitized.

Trigger points can be desensitized in a number of ways. Often through restoring motion to the neck and jaw they become inactive and dissolve. This will be presented in more detail when the use of **physical agents** is discussed. The methods may vary but the results should be the same, i.e. removal of the focus of irritability in the muscle. An excellent reference on **t.p.** therapy or myotherapy (myo meaning muscle) is Pain Erasure, by Bonnie Prudden.

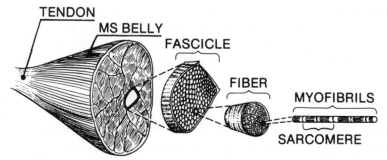

Figure 3. *A muscle belly is composed of bundles of fascicles, which are composed of bundles of fibers, which are composed of bundles of myofibrils. Myofibrils house the smallest units of muscle called sarcomeres. Connective tissue sheaths cover all of the bundles. Near its attachment site the muscle belly ends, and a tendon connects the muscle to the bone. When a muscle contracts a sliding movement occurs within the sarcomeres which shortens the muscle.*

FASCIA

The structure of skeletal muscle is shown in Figure 3. The smallest unit of muscle is the sarcomere. The next largest unit is the myofibril, and increasing in size from that is the muscle fiber, fascicle, and the muscle belly. Muscles are bundles within bundles within bundles of protein surrounded by **connective tissue**. The **connective tissue** component, called **fascia**, surrounds every muscle belly, fascicle, fiber, and myofibril. It both connects and separates structures just like orange sections are enveloped in the separate walls of the orange. The next time you remove the skin from a chicken notice the thin white fibrous sheath that anchors the skin onto the meat. This fibrous sheath is **fascia**. Sometimes **fascia** is thin as in the chicken example and sometimes it is a thick sheath.

There are three divisions of **fascia**. The most superficial layer lies within the skin which in humans is quite thick. The deep **fascia**, which surrounds and courses through and between the muscles, nerves, bones, blood vessels and all of the organs of the body, is the most extensive. The deepest layer of **fascia** which surrounds the brain and spinal cord is referred to as the **dura**. These three divisions house all of the vital tissues of the body, just as thick and thin membranes throughout the orange house the pulp.

The **fascia** spans from the grossest to the finest levels of the body creating a three dimensional web. At the grossest level it becomes a thick sheath, as in the powerful lumbodorsal **fascia** of the low back, serving as protection and support for the muscles of the back. At its finest level, it creates the space for the cells to carry on their processes of energy exchange, respiration, and elimination. Restrictions can be layed down within the **fascia**, due to the mechanical stress of poor posture or trauma, or from chemical changes, as a result of inflammatory processes. These restrictions in the **fascia** can lead to a compromise in any function of the local area or the entire body. The importance of this remarkable system is slowly being recognized. It is an important key in unraveling some of the "mysteries" which surround many chronic pain cases.

Visualize an area of gristle in a piece of meat. In response to trauma or inflammation, the **fascia** can form three dimensional restrictions (gristle) and wrap itself around a nerve or artery or simply restrict the functioning of cells in that area. Remember as a kid trying to pull your fingers out of a Chinese finger trap? The more you pulled the tighter the trap became around your finger. **Fascial** restrictions can exert forces on the body up to 2000 lbs/in^2, which is equivalent to the strength of a radial tire. These restrictions need to be found and released, in order to restore the tissues to their normal functioning. Figure 4 shows how a restriction in the **fascia** can exert a force which can influence the entire body. In this hypothetical example the woman has rounded her shoulders forward slightly in response to a **fascial** restriction. This is only one effect of tight fascia that is observable. The effects on a cellular level as a result of this restriction cannot be seen.

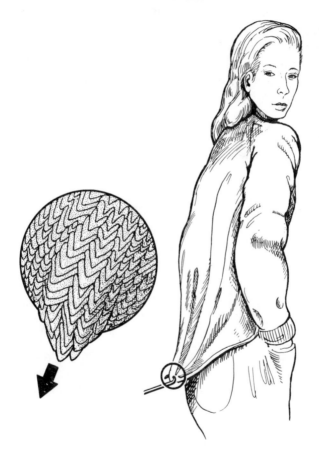

Figure 4. Picture a web of tissue that runs throughout the entire body. When restrictions occur in any part of that web, the entire network is affected, just as a snag in a sweater can distort the entire garment.

This is a relatively new area to be addressed in the profession of physical therapy and so the use of **myofascial release techniques** may not be widespread presently. In time this will be a routine part of treatment.

SUMMARY

Muscle can develop **trigger points** and **fascial** restrictions both of which can be treated with a variety of techniques to desensitize the **trigger points** and release the restrictions. In addition, muscle can become tight and weak. This can be reversed through flexibility and strengthening exercises, recommended at the appropriate time and in the appropriate amount, during the course of treatment.

All muscles in their natural state should be soft and supple. A muscle should inherently be able to generate strong and painfree contractions as well as elongate allowing for flexibility. Even after years of restriction, with proper treatment, muscles can be restored to full functioning. It is a most forgiving and resilient system.

PRINCIPLES OF TREATMENT

REDUCE PAIN AND SPASM. PROMOTE HEALING.

The reason people seek out treatment for their TMJ problem is that they have a complaint, usually pain. So one of the first goals of treatment is to decrease pain. Pain is decreased through reducing **muscle spasm** and promoting healing of the tissues that have been traumatized or have become inflamed. Many modalities are currently available to reduce discomfort, and much of the decision as to which ones will be used is based on what your doctor or therapist feels comfortable administering, as well as which ones yield the best results.

In an **acute** injury to the jaw such as **whiplash** or a blow to the face, there occurs an active **physiological** process where the joint swells, the **muscles spasm** to protect the area, and the tissues become inflamed due to the enormous cellular response, as the area begins to heal itself. Further, the circulation becomes impaired because there is leakage of fluid and cells into surrounding tissue, available oxygen becomes reduced, and energy by-products become built up and do not get carried away through the lymph system which then becomes backed up. If this situation is prolonged it can cause the muscles and joint structures to tighten and restrict motion and lead to the development or activation of **trigger points**, all of which can cause pain.

The **acute** episode usually passes in several days. Treating it at this point helps assure that the problem will not become **chronic**. Chronic pain has been decribed as pain lasting for at least three months. There is another category called **subacute** which refers to a problem between the **acute** and **chronic** stages. To summarize, an **acute** pain is usually a fresh injury. The area may be warm to the touch and swollen. An injury usually stays **acute** for a few days and then moves into the **subacute** phase. If in this phase the tissues do not heal or inflammation does not subside, the problem can become **chronic**. The **chronic** phase can also include pain, inflammation, swelling and **muscle spasm** but the cellular response to attempt to clear the area is much less active than in the **acute** stage. When treatment is begun at this stage, a longer treatment period may be necessary than if it was begun in the **acute** stage. Early intervention is better.

When the inflammatory response stays in the body after the injury or problem heals, the use of **physical agents** can be helpful in reversing this process. **Physical agents** are used to decrease pain, desensitize **t.p.**'s, prepare tissue before stretching or strengthening, and to promote healing. A by-product of decreasing pain is that the quality of the sensory information going back into the **CNS** will be improved which will help break the cycle of pain, spasm, and inflammation. This may explain why the use of **analgesics** alone seem to remedy some problems. Perhaps enough pain relief is achieved to improve the input into the **CNS** and the system corrects itself.

It is often very helpful at this stage of treatment to simultaneously take an **anti-inflammatory** drug. Reducing inflammation through the internal systems of the body as well as through treatment makes good sense. However, one needs to be careful when using pain medications so as not to confuse treatment effects from medication effects. And as was stated in the previous chapter, the use of medication should be monitored carefully by your doctor.

Rest

For an **acute** injury or immediately after surgery of the TMJ, rest or immobilization is the prescribed treatment. Rest of the jaw is difficult but not impossible. A soft diet is recommended as well as the use the of **anti-inflammatory** drugs. A book that you may find helpful at this time is, The Non-Chew Cookbook which is listed in the bibliography in the Resource Section. Another situation which requires rest is an **acute** attack of **gouty arthritis**, which has been reported to occur in the TMJ.

Heat Application

The most common forms of heat used in treating headaches and TMJ are **moist heat packs** and **ultrasound**. **Moist heat packs** (hydrocolator packs) are canvas packs filled with a substance called silica gel, which absorb water. They are placed in a unit which is filled with water and kept at a very high temperature. They are hot enough to burn the skin, and so they are wrapped in several thicknesses of toweling before being placed next to the skin. You can pick up a neck contour pack at the pharmacy for about $12, and use it to heat the jaw and neck areas. But without a heating unit it can be somewhat messy and bothersome. Moist heating pads are more convenient for home use but they do not give quite the same results as **moist heat packs**. The application of **moist heat** to the back, neck and jaw for 20-30 minutes is relaxing for the patient as well as therapeutic for the tissues. I use them with TMJ and headache patients almost all of the time.

If you decide to use **moist heat packs** at home on your own, a few precautions should be noted. If sensation of the skin is not normal, or circulation is impaired for any reason, hot packs should be applied with special care. Use plenty of towels between the skin and the pack and check the area regularly for even and mild reddening. The application of hot packs is safe, when proper safety precautions are taken into account.

Ultrasound is a deep heating agent. Whereas the heat from a hot pack penetrates to a depth of approximately one centimeter, the heat from **ultrasound** penetrates to a depth of five centimeters. So, when you want to heat tissues that lie deep in the body, this is the modality of choice. You may be familiar with the use of **ultrasound** diagnostically in taking pictures of babies while still in the womb. The application used in physical therapy is similar, but a different frequency and technique is used therapeutically to heat the tissues.

The **ultrasound** machine produces high frequency inaudible sound waves by passing an electric current across a crystal. The body absorbs the vibrating sound waves and converts them to heat. It is a safe and effective way to achieve heating of deeper tissues. A conduction gel is used as a medium which allows the **ultrasound** to enter the tissues. **Ultrasound** does not transmit through the air or skin without a medium. The head of the unit is moved around the TMJ for 5-8 minutes. The jaw may be held open through the use of tongue depressors during the treatment to encourage opening. **Ultrasound** can be safely applied to almost any area of the body. See Figure 5.

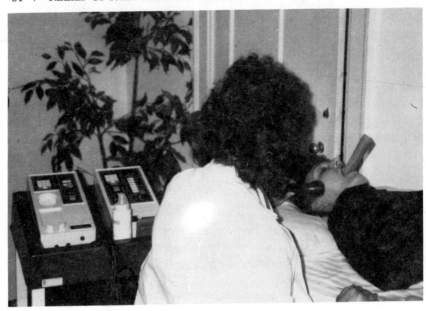

Figure 5. This patient is receiving an ultrasound treatment to the jaw. Stretching can be done simulataneously through the use of tongue depressors inserted between the teeth.

The application of heat results in an increase in local circulation. The benefits of this include the removal of irritating substances, which are present as a result of the inflammatory process. If these are not removed, they can continue to perpetuate the inflammation and pain. Further, when an area is heated, the tissues become more pliable, which allows for greater flexibility. Finally, heating the tissues helps reduce the bombardment of sensory information traveling along the nerves, which helps reduce both pain and spasm.

Ultrasound can also be used to drive **anti-inflammatory** or **analgesic** medication through the skin. This technique is called **phonophoresis**. Common drugs used for this are hydocortisone to stimulate healing and lidocaine to decrease pain. The procedure remains the same. The medication is simply added to the conductive gel.

Cold Application

The two most common uses of **cold therapy** or cryotherapy for headaches and the TMJ, are **cold packs** and **spray and stretch**. The application of **cold packs** for 15-20 minutes reduces swelling, inflammation and **muscle spasm**. First the area undergoes vasoconstriction of the blood vessels. This is followed by vasodiliation, which produces a reddening of the skin. Reddening of the skin as a result of vasodilation can also be observed in heat application. The difference between heat and cold is that cold delivers a greater **counterirritation effect**, which results in numbing of the area. **Counterirritation** means simply supplying a stimulus to the body which the brain pays more attention to. When the stimulation is prolonged less pain is perceived.

Cold is nature's anesthetic. It is often the method of choice for decreasing neck spasm. I have noticed that **cold packs** are not well tolerated on the jaw probably because the face is extremely sensitive. Also some people have difficulty tolerating cold. In order for the application to have the greatest effect, a burning sensation is experienced before the numbing occurs. Therefore, it may not be for everyone.

Cold therapy has been shown to decrease the number of impulses traveling down a nerve which greatly reduces **muscle spasm**. Circulation is also improved as a result of cold application. Temporary joint stiffness is experienced which passes as the tissues warm. Whereas heat application can tend to aggravate many neck problems, ice almost never does. It is best to find which modality works best to alleviate the particular condition. The only rule is to use cold on an **acute** problem. Heat and cold can be interchanged thereafter depending on the preference of the patient and therapist.

Spray and stretch is a technique which is very effective in desensitizing and eliminating **trigger points**. It was first introduced by Dr. Janet Travell. Flourimethane, a vapocoolant spray, is the topical anesthetic most commonly used in this procedure. When this liquid is sprayed on the skin it immediately vaporizes (dries) while freezing the skin. It provides **counterirritation** and increases pain thresholds, so less pain is experienced.

The technique consists of putting the muscle on stretch, and spraying the length of the muscle several times. This is followed by the immediate application of hot packs for 10-15 minutes and then active movement. **Spray and stretch** technique can be applied to any muscle. It works reflexively through the **CNS**, inhibiting the **muscle spasm** and fascilitating the ability of a muscle to elongate or stretch. I use this method of treatment often and find it to be of great value in reducing **muscle spasm**, increasing range of motion, and reducing the sensitivity of **trigger points**. Figure 6 demonstrates **spray and stretch** technique.

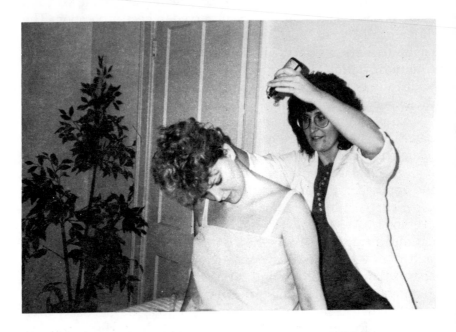

Figure 6. This picture illustrates spray and stretch technique. The entire length of the muscle is sprayed while the muscle is in its fully stretched position. This is an effective treatment technique for releasing tight fascia.

Electrical Stimulation

The thought of someone applying electricity to your body may conjur up fear and images of electrocution. Probably everyone is somewhat apprehensive when it comes to this topic and with good reason. Electricity is that mysterious force that comes out of our walls and the thought of it touching our bodies is not pleasant. And yet most patients once they get used to it actually like and request it.

The use of **electrical stimulation** can be valuable in decreasing pain through its **counterirritation effects**, **anti-inflammatory** effects, and its ability to increase circulation. Several types of **electrical stimulation** devices are available. They are low and high volt generators, **electroacupuncture devices**, and **iontophoretic** devices.

During the treatments, electrodes are prepared with a conductive gel and taped on the body. The electrodes are connected to a machine which delivers a current through the electrodes to the tissue. Treatment times range from 15-30 minutes and can be done for quick pain relief by using a high frequency, or for reduction of swelling and enhancement of healing, by using a low frequency. The high volt devices are somewhat more comfortable than the low volt ones, and so penetration may be deeper since more current can be tolerated. The different frequencies and voltages are simply variations of the same electricity that comes out of the wall socket. Being able to choose how the current gets delivered to the patient gives more treatment options.

An **electroacupuncture device** has a small probe which locates points of decreased skin resistance and then delivers a strong stimulus to the point. This is referred to as noninvasive **acupuncture**, i.e. noninvasive, because electricity is used as the stimulus, as opposed to a needle being inserted into the skin. Areas over inflammed **tendons** and **t.p's**, as well as **acupuncture** points can be stimulated using this device. I do not use these machine personally but my colleagues report good relief of pain particularly in the acute stage of healing. See Figure 7.

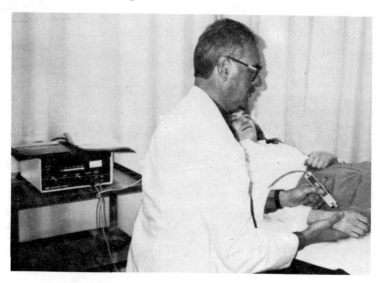

Figure 7. This patient in receiving an electroacupuncture treatment. The probe locates the points to be stimulated and then delivers a strong electrical stimulus to those points. In this picture an acupuncture point is being stimulated in the hand in order to obtain pain relief in the head.

The most common form of **electrical stimulation** used in the treatment of TMJ is **transcutaneous electrical nerve stimulation (TENS)**. When the area is extremely sensitive to touch or the problem is **acute, TENS** is the preferred method of treatment. An added benefit is that many of the units are portable and can be used at home. They can be rented for short term use or bought. The units range in price from $550 to $1200 depending on the number of features. Rentals cost approxmately $125/month. Insurance covers a large percentage of the cost in most cases. See Figure 8.

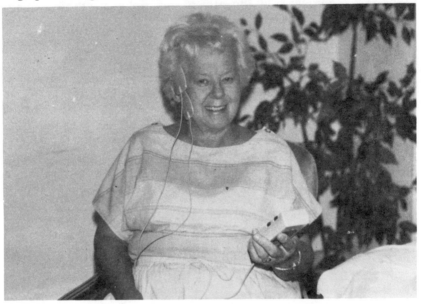

Figure 8. This patient is performing her own TENS treatment. Electrodes are placed on the painful areas and the portable unit, which delivers a comfortable electrical stimulus, is adjusted by the patient.

Similar to **phonophoresis**, where the **ultrasound** drives a drug into the tissues, **iontophoresis** uses **electrical stimulation** to transfer drugs through the skin. Some clinics use this device to drive **analgesics** or **anti-inflammatory** drugs into the TMJ or **trigger points**.

Laser
The use of **lasers** in the treatment of headache and TMJ is gaining in popularity. **Laser** stands for light amplification by stimulated emission of radiation. It is used extensively in surgery and is now

available for therapeutic use. The use of light to promote healing is not new. We have known for a long time that our tissues are light sensitive. In the year 1260 it was reported that Dr. Henri de Mondeville used red light to effectively treat smallpox. The Chinese used light in various forms to treat the body long before that.

People who live in the north report that generally they feel livelier in the summer when it is lighter longer in the day. Dr. Ott, who wrote <u>Health</u> and <u>Light</u>, described a condition of light deprivation long before it was identified more recently by the medical profession. He stated that lack of light can lead to depression and a variety of physical symptoms.

The **laser** delivers a concentrated focus of light in the form of a beam which is aimed at a point on the body and held there for up to several minutes. **Acupuncture** points, **t.p.**'s, or any other points can be stimulated with the **laser** beam. Generally **lasers** are used clinically for pain reduction, and to enhance tissue healing. The mechanisms through which this occurs are not well understood yet. My colleagues who use the **laser** have reported good results, particularly for **acute** problems. See Figure 9.

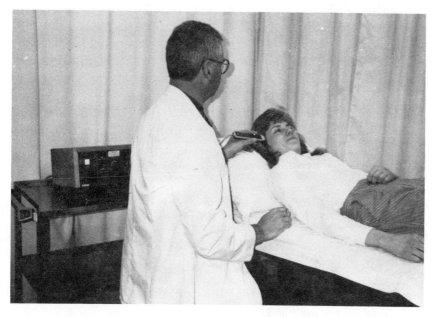

Figure 9. This patient is receiving a laser treatment. The probe is aimed at a point and a beam of light stimulates it. In this picture the TMJ area is being stimulated with the beam of light.

Biofeedback

The use of **biofeedback** in the management of TMJ is included in the **physical agent** section, but it is somewhat different in that no modality is actually applied to the body. **Biofeedback** is used to help someone become aware of tension that they are holding in their muscles and assist them in tension reduction. The theory is that if you can learn to reduce the muscle firing level while using the **biofeedback** equipment, the learned response (relaxation) will carry over into day and night activities. It is commonly used to help control clenching and grinding behavior.

During electromyographic (EMG) **biofeedback** electrodes are placed on a muscle, usually the **masseter**. Other common places to monitor muscle tension are the forehead and the neck. The impulses from the muscle contraction are displayed on a dial where the patient can get a visual readout of the muscle activity and also hear sounds that indicate that the muscles are firing. Through modifying the sound and lowering the readout on the dial, most patients can learn to relax their muscles.

Another common adjunct to EMG **biofeedback** is temperature **biofeedback**. A temperature sensitive probe is placed between the thumb and index finger, and the patient is instructed to raise the temperature at the finger tips. It is thought that people who hold tension in the head and neck tend to pool blood in that area, leaving the fingertips relatively cool. This technique reduces this tendency and improves the overall circulation into the arms. During a biofeedback session, relaxation tapes are often played or the patient is guided through a relaxation exercise by the therapist. See Figure 10.

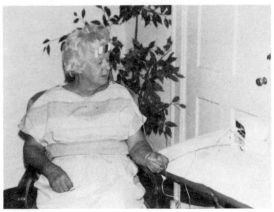

Figure 10. This patient is participating in a biofeedback session. The electrodes on the forehead pick up the electrical activity in the muscles, and display it on a dial, and as a sound. The patient can then learn to lower the reading on the dial, and decrease the sound. In this manner the resting tension level of a muscle can be measured, and the person can learn to decrease the muscle's electrical output, thereby decreasing tension.

SUMMARY

In the **acute** stage of healing the use of **physical agents**, along with rest, are the primary mode of treatment to promote healing. Rest, and the use of physical agents help to reduce pain and **muscle spasm** and decrease swelling. **Subacutely** and **chronically**, modalities are used to prepare the tissues for treatment, such as **myofascial release**, stretch, and/or massage. A wide range of agents is available to choose from, including **moist heat packs, cold packs, spray and stretch, ultrasound, electrical stimulation, laser**, and **biofeedback**. This is useful because often several need to be tried to arrive at the right combination for the particular condition and the particular person.

The use of these modalities can be enormously helpful in pain control, when used appropriately in the hands of skilled clinicians. There is a practice that some professionals are participating in, where unlicensed individuals are being trained on the job to apply modalities to patients. Besides the possibility that in some cases this may be illegal, it is unethical. Someone who administers an **ultrasound** treatment is not necessarily administering physical therapy. The only people who should be administering these modalities are those who are licensed and properly trained to do so.

Physical therapists are one of the licensed professionals who learn the physiology behind the effects of treatment and have a complete understanding of each machine used. Further, there is a thought process determining a particular purpose behind the use of a modality, and an overall plan of treatment that is arrived at through competent training and the experience of practice. You deserve the best!

RESTORING NORMAL RANGE OF MOTION

Every joint has a normal range of motion that it moves through. In Chapter 2 you determined if the range of motion of your jaw was normal by inserting three fingers between your top and bottom teeth. Full range of motion is necessary at every joint in the body for the surrounding tissues of the joint to remain healthy. If your ankle joint became stiff, it would be very noticeable every step you took. But if one of the many small joints of the neck became stiff the other joints around it could compensate for its loss of function. It would be less noticeable to you but equally as serious. The normal functioning of each and every joint of the spine is as important as the normal functioning of the ankle joint. Lack of motion in the cervical spine is one of the most common findings in TMJ.

All **connective tissues** of the body begin deteriorating within hours of immobilization. Tissues need to be stretched throughout their full range of motion regularly to retain their normal properties. **Cartilage** has no blood supply of its own, and receives its nutrients by the loading and unloading which occurs in joints during movement. The well being of all joint structures is dependent upon motion.

It is also necessary for the muscles overlying the joints to allow lengthening to occur freely and easily so that joint motion is not impaired. Just as a tight joint can cause spasming of muscles and activate **trigger points**, an irritated or tight muscle can limit joint range of motion. The two cannot be separated from one another and both must be treated. A complete evaluation of the skeletal system is as important as a complete evaluation of the muscular system. Stiffness of the neck joints, and of the jaw often lead to irritation of the muscles of the neck and the jaw, all of which are common causes of pain associated with TMJ.

Joint Stiffness

The normal range of motion of opening at the TMJ is between 35mm and 50mm. The average range I have observed and try to reestablish is 42-45mm of opening. However, determining what is absolutely normal for that person is somehat subjective. I often ask patients how comfortable opening is for them. There should not be a stiff feeling or pain at the end of the range of normal opening. If there is, I will often persist in gaining a few more millimeters. Establishing normal opening is extremely important so that the tissues surrounding the joint begin to receive the proper stresses, the muscles begin to function normally, and the input into the **CNS** normalizes.

Much of our discussion has focused on the jaw. What is also important in the overall management of TMJ is proper functioning of the cervical spine. V hen we talk about posture and its effects on the head and neck in the next section we will deal with this in much more detail. For right now we will discuss normal mechanics of the cervical spine.

Normal flexion or forward bending of the neck is present when the chin is able to touch the chest. Normal sidebending is present when three fingers can be placed between the tip of the ear and the shoulder, both to the right and left. Normal rotation is present when the chin is in line with the shoulder when you turn to the right and left. Normal extension or backward bending is present when the face is parallel with the ceiling when you look up. If you cannot complete these motions, the joints in your neck have become stiff, or your muscles have become tight and will not allow your neck joints to move. This differentiation can be made by your therapist.

One area that is often neglected is the shoulder. It is an important consideration in TMJ. The TMJ, cervical spine, and shoulder are a closely connected trio and are often involved together. Full elevation of the shoulder can be checked by looking at yourself from the side in the mirror with one arm overhead. Do this one side at a time. Your arm should be in direct line with your body, i.e. 180 degrees from your side. Normal internal rotation is the ability to put your hands up your back almost between your shoulder blades. Do this one side at a time. Normal external rotation is the ability to put your hand on the back of your head, with your elbow out to the side. The shoulder is closely connected biomechanically to the neck. Normal range of motion is important so that the neck does not have to compensate for limited shoulder motion.

There are a number of manual procedures called **joint mobilization techniques** which are effective in freeing the joints. Also, restoring length to the muscles and desensitizing **t.p's**, often result in increased range of motion of the TMJ, neck, and shoulder. What will be discussed next is the treatment of the soft tissues, i.e. the muscles and the **fascia**.

Muscle Tightness

When an area becomes limited in its ability to move, the muscles shorten in response. They can develop **t.p.**'s and taut bands of **connective tissue** within them. Further, the **fascial** sleeve that surrounds and courses through the muscle can bind down like a Chinese finger trap, literally compressing the muscle belly and all its vital structures such as nerves and blood vessels.

The use of **physical agents** alone is not enough to restore normal functioning to a muscle. What is required is good skilled manual techniques in tissue massage and **myofascial release**. The two techniques are not the same and yet you will see the two terms used interchangeably. When done properly, deep massage can do much to open up and free the structures that have been bound down for so long. Through massaging the length of a muscle many of the cross restrictions in a muscle can be freed . Moving across a muscle from side to side can free up many of the restrictions that develop longitudinally in a muscle. Skill is required to feel where the restrictions lie and to know how to restore the area to normal. Many people can be taught how to massage but only a few develop a real sense of the tissue, which is required to make a real change in the tissues.

The **physiological** effects of massage are improved blood flow to the area, relaxation of tissue locally and of the body in general, and improved exchange of nutrients as metabolism improves. Massage also desensitizes areas that are painful so that the **counterirritant effect** of massage leads to pain relief.

The psychological effects of massage are equally as great. We need a great deal of care and understanding when we are in pain and massage can offer much benefit in restoring a feeling of well being. It is easy to pass off massage as not being that important. This is absolutely not the case. Massage is one of the most powerful tools I use to restore an area to normal that has been compromised through trauma or immobility.

After massage, the area immediately softens. The skin color and tone will often change in response to the improvement of circulation. The treatment is extremely enjoyable to the patient. Even if some discomfort is experienced temporarily during massage, people state that it is a "good hurt." Massage may need to be done several times until the body becomes used to its new, relaxed state. It is well worth the time to restore suppleness and length to the muscles. Many people report that much of their mental tension is relieved when the physical tissues are released. More on the body/ mind hook up in Chapter 5.

I am convinced that the single greatest thing that I can do for a patient is to touch them. Massage is one of the mediums I use. And people want to be touched. In some cases they are dying to be touched. I make this statement based on the overwhelming response of the tissues to soften under the hands and the receptivity of the patient to participate in the therapy.

Fascial Tightness

The **fascia** is released through techniques that are similar to massage in that they are manual techniques, but the method of application and their purpose is somewhat different. When the **fascia** binds down it does so three dimensionally, so the restriction needs to be released three dimensionally. It is a very different sensation to get the **fascia** stretched verses the muscle massaged. And although stretching and massaging a muscle does affect some of its **fascial** components, **myofascial release** works specifically on that system of the body. It would be like cutting the lawn with garden shears. The best tool for the job is obviously a lawn mower. And the best tool to restore the **fascia** to normal is **myofascial release**.

This is just one component in the overall treatment plan but it is an important one. This is the most recent technique that I have learned. The results achieved from it, when it is indicated, are often dramatic.

An example will help to clarify just how powerful **fascial** restrictions can be. For several months I had been experiencing a pain in the left side of my neck. Several forms of treatment were tried on my neck to no avail. The pain remained the same. Finally, during an evaluation, a therapist noticed quite a large restriction in my right hamstring in the thigh. The skin overlying the muscle was warm. One session of **myofascial release** to the hamstring eliminated the neck pain. The restriction from the thigh had pulled through the **fascial** sheath and I experienced pain not in the hamstring but in the neck on the opposite side. No one was more astounded than myself. But I learned a valuable lesson, and that is, to evaluate the whole body before I decide where the pain may be coming from.

The superficial **fascia** of the skin and the deep **fascia** of the body are freed through **myofascial release techniques**. The final area where range of motion needs to be restored is in the deepest **fascial** layer called the **dura**. The **dural** restrictions are released through techniques called **craniosacral therapy (CST)**. **CST** is a form of treatment which frees the restrictions that lie within the **cranium** and the spinal canal. These tissues are **Central Nervous System** structures which control the functioning of all the major systems of the body, musculoskeletal, vascular, lymphatic, endocrine, and respiratory. This may explain some of the "strange" and "mysterious" symptoms which are reported by patients, since the dura influences so many of the systems of the body.

In the early 1900's, Dr. William Sutherland, an osteopathic physician, discovered a circulatory system within the **cranium** (head) and down through the spine that operated independent of the heart and lung systems. The fluid that is present within this chamber is called cerebrospinal fluid. Cerebrospinal fluid bathes the **Central Nervous System** structures and supplies nutrients to the tissues. It is pumped at a rate of 6-12 times per minute throughout this closed system. This pumping action is created by the expansion and contraction within the **cranium**, and an up and down movement at the end of the spine, the sacrum, where the **dura** ends.

What is taught at most medical and dental schools is that the 28 bones of the skull are fused and do not move. Dr. Sutherland suggested that the **cranium** is a collection of rhythmically moveable bones, and that the **craniosacral** system "provides the internal milieu for the development, growth and functional efficiency of the brain and spinal cord from the time of embryonic formation to death.* According to **CST** normal movement of the **cranium** and the sacrum is critical.

The **dura** is essentially the covering of the brain, the tissue between the **sutures** (joints) of the skull, and the covering of the spinal cord with all of its nerve roots. It is embedded within the deep **fascia** of the body. Restrictions in the **fascia** anywhere in the body, can pull through to the **dura** (as gristle courses through a piece of meat), and cause many symptoms, including TMJ and headache. The three **fascial** layers, the superficial layer of the skin, the deep layer of the body, and the **dura** of the **craniosacral** system, are intimately related. The viewing of the body in this more "whole" way takes us far beyond viewing the TMJ as an isolated joint in the face. The **mandible** is dependent on a normal relationship and

*taken from Craniosacral Therapy by Upledger and Vredevoogd

freedom of movement between all of the cranial bones. After all, the **mandible** along with the **fossa** of the **temporal bone**, comprises the TMJ itself.

The bones of the **cranium** are shown in Figure 11. All of the bones are treated in **CST** including the sacrum at the the lower end of the spine. In TMJ, restriction is most prevalent in the **mandible** moving off of the **temporal bone**, and the **temporal bone** moving between the parietal, sphenoid, and occipetal bones.

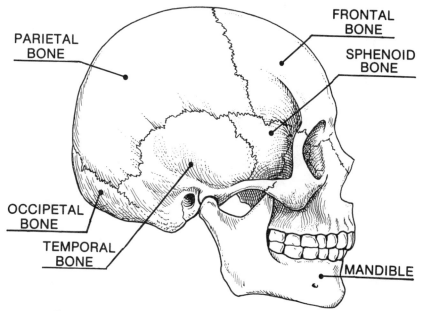

Figure 11. The bones of the skull are joined at the sutures and at the TMJ. The flat bones of the skull form the vault for the brain. The facial bones form the supporting structure for the face.

The techniques of **CST** consist of light pressures on the bones in the direction necessary to free the restriction. There are practitioners who study this system for many years and use these techniques exclusively. It has been a highlight of my career to begin to develop an understanding of this most fascinating system. This is a controversial area but one that is gaining much attention in medical, dental, and physical therapy circles. The controversy exists around whether the **sutures** do indeed move, and the explanation of the mechanism through which it works. More research is clearly needed in this area. **CST** is another example of a technique which is not for everyone for every problem. But when it is indicated, the results are often dramatic. Many chronic, difficult cases of TMJ and headaches respond well to **CST**.

IMPROVE POSTURE

When you were a child and your grandmother yelled at you to stand up straight she was handing out a good piece of advice. We slumped for good reasons, because no one understood us, our breasts budded too soon or too abundantly (as was the case for me), or we were just plain lazy. As we got older we carried loads of books and sat at desks for longer and longer periods of time. As we got older still we became more sedentary and got desk jobs. We sit in our cars going to work, and while home we become potatoes on the couch.

All of these activities, as well as most of the sports we engage in, require the head and arms to be positioned in front of our bodies for extended periods of time. If the opposite group of muscles is not strengthened, and if the muscles in constant use are not stretched, the body will tend to become imbalanced over time. This needs correction. A forward head and rounded shoulders are thought to be a significant contributing factor in headache and TMJ.

Further, a habit that some people develop is open mouth breathing. Open mouth breathing is an abnormal breathing pattern that can develop in response to an abnormal tongue position or **chronically** blocked nasal passages. The normal breathing pattern consists of taking air in and out through the nose. In this way, the nose functions to warm and filter the air before it enters the lungs. When the air enters the lungs, the **diaphragm**, which is the primary muscle of breathing, descends, which allows the lungs to fully expand. This means that the chest should not rise and fall during breathing, but rather the abdomen should go out as you inhale, and in as you exhale.

Notice two things about your breathing. Are you breathing through your nose, and are you using your **diaphragm** to breath? If your tongue is in its proper resting position you will automatically be breathing through your nose. Next, notice if your abdomen moves up and down when you breathe, which indicates that you are using your **diaphragm**. If you are not using your **diaphragm**, you will first have to make yourself aware of that fact, and then, you will need to learn how to use it.

If you have determined that you are not using your **diaphragm** (because when you observe yourself inhaling your chest rises instead of your abdomen protruding), the following exercise will help you to change your breathing pattern. Sit comfortably in a chair. Place one hand on your chest and one hand on your abdomen. Look at your hands. When you inhale your top hand should not move, and your bottom hand should be pushed away from the body. The **diaphragm** drops as you inhale and the abdominal contents get pushed out slightly, which is why your bottom hand moves. As you breathe out, your bottom hand moves back toward the body, while your top hand still remains quiet.

Your awareness during the day of breathing through the nose and breathing with the **diaphragm** will help in reversing the two unhealthy habits which often accompany TMJ. Figure 12 shows a picture of the **diaphragm** during breathing. The **diaphragm** is the muscle that is primarily responsible for breathing. When we use it, we use fewer of the accessory muscles of breathing. Breathing in this way is effortless. It may take some practice, but this nasal-diagphragmatic breathing pattern is what your body was **physiologically** designed to do. Within a short time this will feel normal to you.

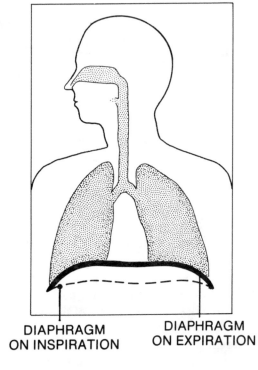

DIAPHRAGM
ON INSPIRATION

DIAPHRAGM
ON EXPIRATION

Figure 12. The diaghragm is the primary muscle of breathing. As you breath in, it descends, and as you breath out, it rises.

You have probably noticed that when you have a cold and your nose is blocked that it is difficult to breathe. Some people breathe through their mouth routinely and are unaware of this abnormal pattern that they have developed. Further, when the upper chest is used to breathe, accessory muscles become the primary muscles of breathing instead of the **diaphragm**. This alters the normal functioning of this area. When the normal **physiology** of breathing is altered, the energy cost to the body increases.

Now that you have a sense of what the normal breathing pattern should be let's elaborate on some other points, since this is so important. Next, count how many breaths you take per minute. One cycle would be considered an inspiration and an expiration. A normal rate is approximately twelve breaths per minute. I have found that most people breathe faster than that, which is abnormal. I breathe four times per minute. That means that I breathe three times more efficiently than normal. I attribute this to the relaxation techniques that I have used and continue to use everyday. There is room for variation here, but you should use twelve breaths per minute as a general guideline. Next, notice if you spend the same amount of time taking air in as you do letting it out. Inspiration should be equally as long as expiration. The quality of the movement should be smooth, i.e. no jerkiness throughout inspiration or expiration. There should be no pauses between breaths or at the end of inspiration. Finally, breathing should be quiet. There should be no noise when the air is moving in and out.

General relaxation of the body has been strongly correlated with proper breathing. When breathing is slow, deep, diaphragmatic, regular, smooth, and quiet, the body can attain a relaxed state. When the breathing is shallow, quick, irregular, or noisy, the body cannot relax. The next time that you become aware that you are tense, notice what happens to your breathing. You may hold your breath or breathe more shallowly when you are standing in line, writing a check, or on hold on the phone. When you notice this, change it. Reestablish deep, smooth, regular, quiet breathing whenever you can remember to do so. Spend some time practicing this while you are in as relaxed a state as possible to give yourself the feeling of what " normal" is. It will be much easier to reestablish this new pattern the more familiar it is to you. As you begin to gain some awareness and control over this important **physiological** function, you will have at your fingertips an incredible tool that can help you to establish and maintain relaxation of the body. And now, back to our discussion on forward head posture.

Some of us may be genetically predisposed to developing a forward head while others of us may develop one in response to environmental/lifestyle factors described previously. And some may develop one as a result of changing the way in which they breathe. A forward head is an extremely prevalent postural pattern that people develop. It needs correction!

Ideal postural alignment is presented in Figure 13. An example of forward head posture (FHP) is given in Figure 14. Not only is the head forward in Figure 14, the upper back is rounded and the low back has an exaggerated curve. It is also possible for the low back to flatten in response to a forward head. Misalignment can begin in any area of the body and result in a forward head. Almost no one aligns perfectly with the **postural plumb line**, but we should come close. The body is adaptable, and yet, when we reach the end of our adaptable limit we can begin to develop symptoms.

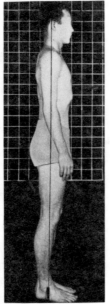
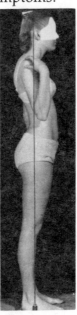

Figure 13. This depicts a person in ideal alignment with the postural plumb line. Think of the balance that is required of the muscles in the front and back of the body to allow such alignment. (left)

Figure 14. This depicts typical forward head posture with a rounded upper back and increased curve in the low back. (right)

Reproduced by permission from, Muscles: Testing and Function, by Florence Kendall and Elizabeth McCreary, editor, Baltimore, Williams and Wilkins Co, 1983.

The following is a proposed chronology of events that occurs as the head begins to move forward. The curve in the low back becomes more exaggerated or straighter, either of which can lead to degeneration of the joints and discs of the lower back. Further, the muscles of the low back have to work harder to hold the body upright because there is this "bowling ball" (the head) hanging out in front of the body instead of positioned over the body. As the head comes forward, to keep the eyes level with the horizon the head gets tilted back on the neck which compresses the suboccipetal muscles at the base of the skull. See Figure 15. Compression of these muscles and of the **occipetal nerve**, which actually pierces through one of the neck muscles, is one of the most common causes of headache.

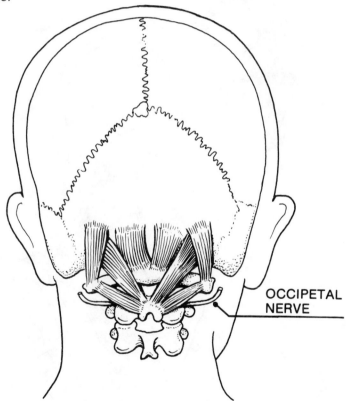

OCCIPETAL
NERVE

Figure 15. The suboccipetal muscles are small muscles deeply set in the upper posterior neck. They rotate and backward bend the head on the neck. The occipetal nerve is shown in relation to these muscles. This nerve actually pierces through one of the neck muscles in the layer just above this one.

Due to the position of the head being forward, the muscles in the back of the neck shorten and tighten. See Figures 16 and 17. Notice the extensiveness of the posterior musculature. These are thick layers of large muscles some of which run the length of the entire

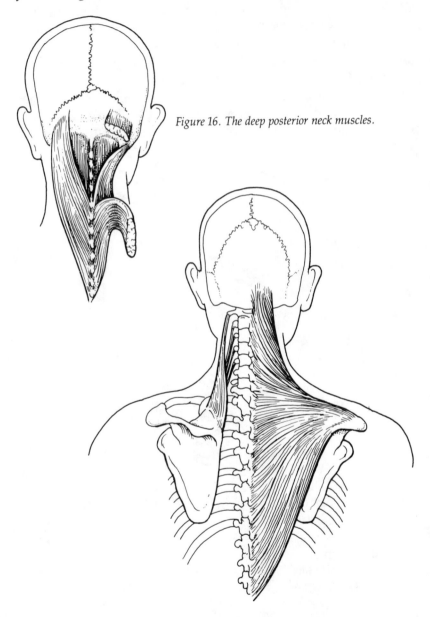

Figure 16. The deep posterior neck muscles.

Figure 17. The superficial posterior neck muscles.

spine, some which end at the mid back, and some which end at the base of the neck. Normal length needs to be restored to the group of posterior neck muscles. The muscles in the front and side of the neck become overly active and the hyoid bone is usually elevated. See Figure 18.

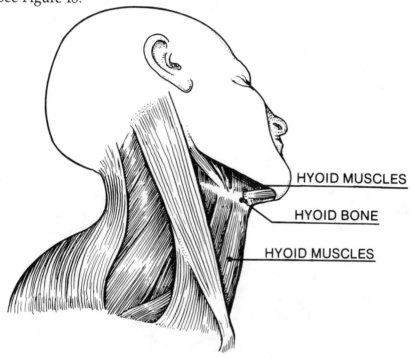

HYOID MUSCLES

HYOID BONE

HYOID MUSCLES

Figure 18. The anterior and lateral neck muscles.

Notice again the massive musculature and how intricately related these muscles must be to one another. The hyoid bone is a free floating bone dependent upon a balance between the muscles above and below it. Can you see how important it is for these great muscle masses, the flexors in front of the neck, and the extensors in back of the neck, to have proper length and strength? The improper position of the head on the neck, and the improper position of the neck on the body, changes the normal relationship that these structures have with one another, and can lead to a variety of symptoms. PROBLEMS WITH THE MUSCLES OF THE NECK AND JAW ARE THE MOST COMMON CAUSES OF TMJ.

Another change that often occurs in forward head posture is elevation of the first rib. When the first rib elevates, the major blood vessels and nerves that go to the arm can become compressed. This can account for pain which is experienced down the arm. Further, poor posture, including rounding of the shoulders and the mid back results in a decreased lung capacity. If you are not breathing as deeply, you are not oxygenating your tissues as well. Finally, the **mandible** is pulled back due to the tension on the tissues of the neck from the head being forward. This results in an altered position for the muscles of chewing, an altered tooth contact pattern, and altererd TMJ mechanics.

All of this sounds terrible but there is good news. It is quite easy, with the help of a willing subject, to change a forward head. And after reading about all of the benefits that you can receive from making this improvement, I would guess that you would be willing to do a couple of things to help turn this around.

Your therapist needs to release the tightness in the **fascia** and muscles in the back of your neck. You can help keep the length of the posterior structures, through stretching, which should be taught to you individually. A stretch that is helpful in maintaining length is demonstrated in Figure 19. When the posterior neck mus-

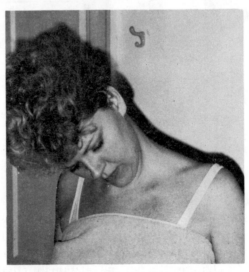

Figure 19. Drop your head forward and to the side and let the weight of your head stretch the back of your neck. Stretch for at least 90 seconds.

cles shorten they cause the head to backward bend on the neck. By restoring proper length posteriorly, the head is able to assume a more upright position. If length is not restored, the head literally cannot move back. This is very important!

Restoring strength to the neck muscles is as important as restoring proper length. In a forward head posture just as the muscles in back of the neck tend to develop tightness, the muscles in front of the neck tend to be weak. The anterior neck muscles need to be strengthened so that they can hold the head upright in good alignment.

An exercise which is used to improve the overall posture will now be presented. It is called the Wall Exercise and was proposed by Florence Kendall, a highly respected physical therapist, who's life work is in the area of muscle and posture. When performed correctly this exercise works every muscle which holds us up against gravity. Do not be deceived. This is a very difficult and powerful exercise. Some of the best weight lifters at the club where I work out cannot do even one of these properly because their bodies are so imbalanced.

The beauty of this exercise is that it works the anterior neck, upper back and lower abdominals at the same time, as well as stretches the back of the neck and low back. So many exercises have us just work one muscle or group of muscles at a time. We use all of these muscles dynamically, not one at a time. This exercise most closely approximates how we use our muscles functionally in our everyday activities. Begin slowly and build your endurance. When I first learned this exercise five years ago I could not complete one repetition. Now I do 30-40 without stopping. When you feel you are ready to strengthen even more, you may add three to five pound weights in your hands. Figure 20 & 21 demonstrates the wall exercise.

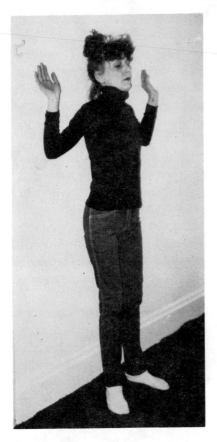

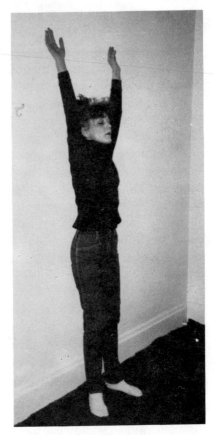

Figure 20. The wall exercise, starting position. Place your back, head, elbows and hands against the wall, heels 3" from wall. Flatten your low back against the wall by contracting your abdominal muscles and pulling in your belly. Breathe normally.

Figure 21. Raise the arms as high as you can while keeping everything next to the wall and your back flat against the wall. Then, lower your arms slowly. The exercise consists of slowly raising and lowering your arms.

NEUROMUSCULAR REEDUCATION

So now you know the many important reasons why the head needs to be positioned correctly on the body. You also know an exercise, the wall exercise, which strenghtens the antigravity muscles, which will help you maintain a more upright posture. And you now know that nasal-diaghragmatic breathing conserves energy through eliminating the use of accessory muscles and allows for greater use of your lung tissue. There are two more important factors to be considered in restoring normal function to this area, and those are resting tongue position and swallowing.

Notice where the tip of your tongue is positioned in your mouth. Most people say it is behind the bottom front teeth. It should be behind the top front teeth. When you say the word "in" your tongue is at rest. Take a moment to refer to Figure 7 of Chapter 2, which reviews the resting position of the tongue. This position needs to be maintained except during the activities of eating or talking. Being aware during the day of proper tongue position helps to restore normal function to the area and relieves strain on the muscles of the jaw.

The tongue is the most powerful force in the mouth. It's proper position is important for maintenance of the normal position of all the cranial bones as well as maintenance of normal posture of the neck. Another reason for maintaining this position is to minimize problems with swallowing.

Swallowing is often a problem for people with TMJ. Swallowing is a highly coordinated activity dependent upon a balanced musculature. When imbalances are present, such as those seen in forward head posture, difficulty in swallowing can occur. This can take the form of an anterior tongue thrust during swallowing. In an anterior tongue thrust, every time swallowing occurs the tongue pushes forward against the teeth. This needs correction because it is an abnormal pattern which strains the tissues.

Swallowing should be effortless. If swallowing is difficult or painful, you need proper instruction in the correct sequence of swallowing. This needs to be done one on one with the therapist. This instruction, along with improving posture and tongue position, will contribute greatly to improving the overall functioning of the entire head and neck area.

Exercise

This section describes a set of exercises recommended for use in TMJ. It is called the 6X6 program and was originally proposed by Mariano Rocabado, a physical therapist, who is noted for his extraordinary work in the area of TMJ. I teach these exercises to all of my patients and streamline them to suit the individual. Six repetitions of six exercises are completed six times daily. They serve three purposes. The first is that they get the person involved in their own care. The second is that the person begins to develop an awareness of the functioning of the area. And thirdly, the exercises gradually and gently stress and strenghten the jaw which promotes healing.

These exercises need to be prescribed individually. All of these exercises are not for everyone. Some people who read this book may not have access to a health care practitioner who can teach these exercises to them. So I am presenting them, but I do not recommend doing them without supervision from a trained health professional. If you begin to do these exercises and they increase pain, decrease the amount of exercise or stop exercising. They can be done in any position. However, I prefer sitting. All six exercises are done six times daily, six repetitions each exercise. Each exercise is done slowly, smoothly, and gently.

The first exercise reinforces the resting position of the tongue. Place the tip of the tongue behind the top front teeth and make a clock sound with your tongue, where the jaw opens slightly. This exaggeration helps sensitize the area and gets your palate used to the tongue being there. Also, a gentle downward force is delivered to the jaw when you make this sound, which has a relaxing effect on the jaw.

The second exercise is controlled opening. Place the tip of your tongue on the roof of your mouth, in the center of your mouth. Now, open and close as far as you can comfortably, without causing pain, and without your tongue dropping down. Keeping the tongue up, limits the amount of forward **glide** at the joint surface, and encourages rotation or **rolling** at the TMJ. This helps in pain control in many cases. This is a good and gentle exercise for the jaw.

The third exercise strengthens and improves coordination of the muscles of the jaw. It is called rhythmic stabilization, and the muscles of the jaw must contract to stabilize the joint. With the tongue in resting position, gently resist all motions of the jaw with your hands; opening, closing, side glide left, and side glide right. Resist the motion with your hands. Feel the contraction of the muscle but do not allow the jaw to actually move. This is an **isometric contraction**.

Do not resist too hard. Just a strong but easy painfree contraction achieves the best result. More is not better here. When you get really good at becoming aware of and controlling the contractions you can even resist in diagonals. This one takes the most amount of concentration and should first be learned in front of a mirror where you can observe your jaw resisting the movement. See Figure 22.

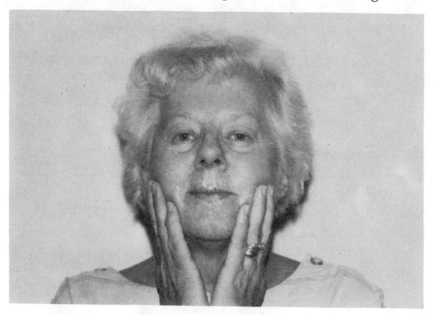

Figure 22. Rhythmic Stabilization. Resist all motions gently.

The fourth exercise improves range of motion in the upper neck joints. Place both hands with your fingers interlaced behind your head. Drop your head forward on your neck and then bring your head back on yor neck as far as you can without causing pain. Move very slowly. It is not intended for the neck to move on the body but rather the head to move up and down on the neck. See Figure 23.

The fifth exercise is called axial extension and is meant to reverse forward head (as does the wall exercise). Tuck your chin and lift your chest. It is helpful to picture someone pulling up and back on a string at the top of your head. A mistake often made is that people tip their heads back instead of tucking the chin and elongating the neck. Refer back to Figures 13 & 14 and note the difference in the position of the head in both photographs.

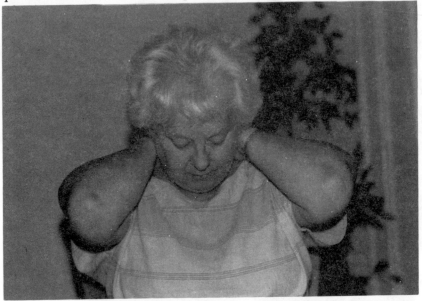

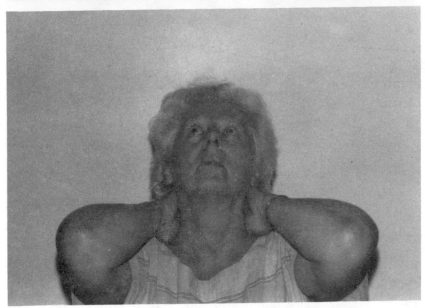

Figure 23. *Upper Cervical Range of Motion. Clasp both hands behind the neck. Nod forward, and then tilt your head back, as far as you can comfortably.*

The sixth and final exercise is called shoulder retraction and consists of dropping the shoulders and pinching the shoulder blades together. This counteracts the tendency most of us have to carry the shoulders high and to round them forward which moves the shoulder blades out.

These exercises need to be demonstrated and streamlined for you. When you have pain and dysfunction, the normal feedback mechanisms from the brain to the muscles are altered and you need verbal, and touch feedback from the therapist, as well as visual feedback from your own image in the mirror, to correct the movement dysfunctions of the TMJ. I present these exercises because they are the classic ones prescribed for TMJ, and exercise is a key element in the overall recovery. Once learned they are easily carried out during the day. You might want to make a list of the exercises on a card and keep it around where it can serve as a reminder for you to do them. The exercises are:

Rest Position of the Tongue and Mandible "In"
Control of TMJ Rotation
Rhythmic Stabilization of the TMJ
Upper Neck Range of Motion
Axial Extension of the Cervical Spine
Shoulder Girdle Retraction

I like to combine the last two, so when you elongate the spine and tuck the chin you drop the shoulders and pinch the shoulder blades together. I then make the sixth exercise six nasal-diaghragmatic breaths. This reinforces the correct breathing pattern and relaxes the body.

Additional stretches or exercises for the neck or other areas of the body may be indicated. These will be recommended on an individual basis by your therapist. The more you can reinforce all during the day what is being gained in therapy, the greater will be the results.

Exercise needs to be graded and introduced at the approriate time in treatment. This is the single greatest factor along with reinjury that produces setbacks in therapy. Too much too soon is not good. Eventually, exercise helps restore an area to normal, but if begun too soon, it can cause more irritation and pain. In the course of treatment, as pain begins to subside, exercise should be introduced and modified, based on how the tissues respond and how the patient responds.

BODY MECHANICS AND AWARENESS

The more you can become aware of the habits that may contribute to your problem, the greater will be your gains. For example, three half hour therapy treatments per week will not reverse the effects of five hours of gum chewing per day. Other common habits are pen and pencil chewing, clenching the jaw, and holding the head up by resting your chin on your hands. Try to become aware during the course of your day what habits you have developed that could be contributing to stressing this area. This will require some attention but it is well worth it. One of my patients reported to me that one day he became aware that when he wrote, he tilted his head to the left. Correcting this habit did have an effect on the amount of tension that he felt in the left side of his neck.

Sometimes it is necessary to decide what you are willing to give up in order to get better, and how willing you are to participate in your treatment. I get people actively involved because I know that is the only way to get lasting results. There isn't a person on this planet who hasn't wished they could take a pill to make a problem go away. Awareness, determination, and patience get you better, and that takes time and effort on your part. One moment of impatience can strain the tissues. Being aware is a full time job and if you are in pain it is your most important full time job. No one can do this for you. Decide that you are going to give your body what it needs.

The following is general information on good body mechanics. It would be a good practice for you to begin to notice how you are holding your body when you move and go about your activities. Do you hold items that you are lifting close to your body and do you lift with the legs? Do you stand on a stool to move things to high places so that you do not have to raise your arms too high? Begin to think about how you can make tasks easier for yourself.

Standing on a ladder is difficult for anyone with a spine problem, particularly the low back. This is because the support under the feet is so poor. Try to avoid this altogether. Sweeping, vacuuming, and snow shoveling cause the spine to twist. These three activities tend to aggravate the low back greatly and can contribute to irritating a neck or jaw problem. They can be done without twisting but you have to be creative. Use a push broom to sweep, push the vacuum with both hands, and face the snow bank and throw the snow in front of you while shoveling. Changing how you do these activities, can decrease the amount of rotation of the spine, which can decrease the strain placed upon it.

Sitting is a particular problem because most chairs and car seats do not support the lumbar curve. Rather, they tend to flatten the back, which contributes to forward head posture as well as ligamentous strain of the low back. I suggest the use of a lumbar cushion for all headache and TMJ patients. They are an invaluable aid and incredibly comfortable. Even though they appear to be more appropriate for low back problems their use is just as necessary for neck and jaw problems, because the low back is the base upon which the neck functions. Low back cushions help relieve low back strain and decrease forward head posture. If you will be sitting for extended periods, and we all do, get one of these.

The use of a cervical pillow for sleeping can be helpful. There are many on the market. They are designed to support the natural curve in the neck and relieve pressure on the face in the sidelying position. I find them to be infinitely more comfortable than a regular pillow. But you have to try these for yourself. Some patients tell me that they unconsciously throw them across the room in the middle of the night! Your comfort is the most important factor. If you are happy with your pillow keep it. If you wake up in the morning with a tight neck, more pain, or are sensitive to pressure on your face, consider changing to a cervical pillow.

These little accessories make life easier. Insurance covers most of them. All lumbar cushions and cervical pillows feel different. Find the ones that fit your body the best and are the most comfortable to you.

Anyone who has a desk job needs an adjustable chair with arm rests. The most important adjustment is the height of the chair in relation to the desk top. This is an individual adjustment. The ideal height is one where your shoulders are positioned in front of your body at an angle of 25 degrees and out to the side of your body at an angle of 15 degrees. In this position the muscles of the neck and shoulders are the most relaxed. Also, have your lumbar support in your chair and get up hourly to move around. If you absolutely cannot get another chair, scout the office for one that feels the best for you. A good office chair costs less than $100. If you think this is an unrealistic request, I ask you to think again. This is your only body. If you sit all day, why wouldn't you pay special attention to your chair?

Working on a computer terminal strains the eyes as well as the shoulders and neck but here are a few suggestions to minimize the strain. Make sure that the keyboard is placed so that the angle of your shoulder is as stated above, slightly forward, and out to the side. Keeping the monitor low so that it is at, or slightly below eye level, decreases eye and neck strain. Periodically stretch your whole body forward in the chair with your arms out straight. Performing slow neck circles is helpful. Every hour look away from the screen for several minutes. Do another activity for that period of time. Holding reading material too close, or looking too closely at the monitor, contributes to eye strain and headache. The ideal reading distance is 12-15 inches.

Becoming aware of clenching or grinding behavior is the first step in reducing its occurence. During the day, notice if a coping technique you use is to clench the jaw. You might be surprised to find yourself doing this. The more aware of this you can become, the more you will be able to let that habit go. Night clenching is more difficult to control because you are in an altered state of awareness. **Biofeedback** may be promising for you in decreasing clenching behavior.

Lifting heavy objects strains the neck. Try to avoid this altogether. When carrying a shoulder bag, become aware of how you carry that shoulder. Remind yourself to relax that shoulder and to let that side of your body move freely. Shoes that give minimal support, such as sandals, or precarious support, such as high heels, alter the foundation for the spine. Shoes with a wide base of support and a good sole, which absorbs shock, are recommended. There are some good quality stylish shoes on the market. Crossing the legs for long periods while sitting strains the back and is not good for the circulation. Shifting your weight from one side to the other while standing contributes to weakness of the hip musculature. Standing on concrete floors is a great strain on the entire body. Most stores have a thin piece of linoleum over concrete which is just as hard. Stand on a cushioned mat or wear Sorbathane inserts in your shoes.

Sorbathane is a substance developed by Nike which absorbs a large amount of compressive force, which gets transmitted up the leg and through the spine, during activities such as standing, walking, or running. The use of inserts while engaging in any activity which requires prolonged or excessive weight bearing will greatly decrease the amount of strain on the musculoskeletal system.

There may be other habits or activities you engage in which are unique to your lifestyle that may be perpetuating your problem. It would be worth your time and effort to think about this. I can give you an example of an awareness that I had about one year ago.

While writing I began to notice how tense I held my neck and arm. I remembered that in penmanship class in the fifth grade the nun used to walk up and down the aisle, and would hit us over the back of the hand with a ruler if she caught us with our eyes off of our paper. At age 35 I was perpetuating the experience that I had when I was ten years old, of writing in fear, and holding my body stiff. I was still preparing to get whacked. Having had that awareness, I can now consciously relax while I write and remind myself that no one is going to smack the back of my hands. This may appear absurd to some but these early experiences can have a powerful influence on people's lives. See what you can discover about your habit patterns and begin to break them through conscious awareness.

SUMMARY

Physical therapy promotes healing by reducing pain and decreasing muscle spasm. Freeing the joints and restoring length to the muscles and fascia, restores normal range of motion. Exercise improves strength and helps restore an area to normal. Improving the posture minimizes the stress that is placed on the tissues. By tuning into how we move, how we hold our bodies when we move, and our general habits and behaviors, and then changing them, we can remove some of the perpetuating factors in pain production. Paying attention to all of these factors contributes to reestablishing normal function and the elimination of pain.

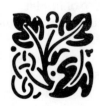

The
Inner
You

To begin with, you've got to understand that a seagull is an unlimited idea of freedom, an image of the Great Gull, and your whole body, from wingtip to wingtip, is nothing more than your thought itself.

— Richard Bach
Johnathan Livingston Seagull

nd a woman spoke, saying, tell us of pain.
And he said:

> Your pain is the breaking of the shell that encloses your understanding.
> Even as the stone of the fruit must break, that its heart may stand in the sun, so must you know pain.
> And could you keep your heart in wonder at the daily miracles of your life, your pain would not seem less wonderous than your joy;
> And you would accept the seasons of your heart, even as you have always accepted the seasons that pass over your fields.
> And you would watch with serenity through the winters of your grief.
> Much of your pain is self-chosen.
> It is the bitter potion by which the physician within you heals your sick self.
> Therefore trust the physician, and drink his remedy in silence and tranquility:
> For his hand, though heavy and hard, is guided by the tender hand of the Unseen.
> And the cup he brings, though it burn your lips, has been fashioned of the clay which the Potter has moistened with His own sacred tears.

— Kahil Gibran

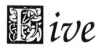

Five

INTRODUCTION

There is a world inside of you that only you know about. There are places within the recesses of your mind where only you can go...alone...with no one else. With no one else we go to these places, to think, to feel, to dream and sometimes to hurt. For some people this inner space may be a familiar sanctuary. For others, it may seem strange ground. For others still, it may be territory to be avoided.

Whether your inner space is terra firma, quicksand, or a big black hole, nevertheless, it is your space. And this is where we begin to unravel this thing that we are calling your pain. Throughout your experience you will no doubt run the gammut of emotions. You will at times feel out of control. You will wonder if you can make it. Perhaps you will even give thought to ending it all. Know that all of these feelings are natural. Know that you are not alone in your experience. And know that it can pass.

Physical pain cuts deeper than the body. It pierces past the mind. It burrows into the soul. Pain changes everything. You can forget who you are with pain. But the real you is in there waiting. You must have faith. You cannot give up on yourself.

The physical pain that you experience indicates that something is wrong. Through the knowledge gained from reading this book, you can now locate the right people to help find the problem and solve it. Much suffering comes from doubt and confusion, doubt about the prescribed treatment, and confusion about what to do. That is why you must find competent professionals, so that the pressure to solve the problem is off of you. You will have plenty of work to do to enhance the therapy. If you do the outer work of finding good doctors and therapists, and the inner work which is what this chapter is about, you can become painfree in time. The body can heal. You can be well again.

In the last chapter we talked about how to fix the body. But the body isn't in this by itself. It is powerfully influenced by the mind. In this chapter we are going to focus on how the body and mind are connected, how they influence each other, and how we can use that connection to our advantage.

Perhaps there are some people who do not feel the need to analyze, probe, or think about this. That is fine. Those people can skip this chapter. But for those individuals who want to make some sense out of the experiences life hands them, and for those who want to use all of the tools available to them to improve, I invite you to read on. For although it is not for everyone, a life examined is surely a richer and deeper one.

THE MIND/BODY CONNECTION

The mind exists within the physical structure of the brain. The brain, with its billions of nerve connections throughout the entire body, is deeply embedded in the body's tissues. The mind, which for purposes of discussion we are calling the brain, is so closely interconnected with the body that it is difficult if not impossible to separate the two. A great deal of research on the effect of the mind on the body is being conducted around the world. These studies are now verifying what many scientists and behaviorists have long suspected, that the mind exerts powerful influences over the body.

When the mind senses danger, whether real or imagined, the body responds by heightening all of its functions. **Adrenalin** is pumped into the system, which allows us to mobilize quickly so that we can get to safety. We call this the **flight-fight** response, which prepares us either to run, or stay and defend ourselves. This is a primitive reflex, appropriate for short term coping and for real dangers, but wearing on the system when the response becomes prolonged or in response to imagined danger. Our complicated lives sometimes require us to defend ourselves and justify our existence in this world, which can keep us in this "ready" state. Worry, anxiety, and fear also keep us in this state. One technique already mentioned, which can help reverse this **physiological** response, is nasal-diaphragmatic breathing. Breathing deeply, regularly, smoothly, quietly, and with no pauses helps restore relaxation to the body. Other relaxation and coping techniques are offered in the books that will be presented next.

What we are learning is that the body is physically altered in response to the inner workings of our minds. The thoughts we think, and the beliefs that we hold are not abstractions. They trigger electrical and chemical events in areas of the brain which control every bodily function. This is a most exciting area in which work in many disciplines is being reported in its respective literatures.

A rich network of blood vessels was discovered in the brain which links the hypothalamus, the main regulator of the body, to the pituitary, the master gland. It was found that certain substances travel down these blood vessels, from the hypothalamus to the pituitary, which cause different reactions in the body, depending upon our mental state. These substances, as well as blood flow and other parameters can be measured. The following is a summary of what we have learned about how our emotional state affects the physiology of our bodies.

The presence of excessive stress hormones in the blood, which are present when we are under stress, gives rise to artery damage, and higher cholesterol and uric acid levels. The elevation of these two substances, cholesterol and uric acid, has been linked to heart disease. In addition, antibody and killer T cell actvity diminishes in the presence of excessive stress hormone, both of which are necessary to keep immunity high. Diminished concentration or activity of T cells or antibodies results in lower immunity to infections of all kinds. The saliva of students who were taking examinations was tested for the presence of certain antibodies. It was found that the concentration of antibodies which help fight colds was decreased. This helps explain why colds are so prevalent around exam time. Antibody and killer T cells also act to suppress tumor formation. In this way, abnormally high cell growth is kept in check by the body. A decrease in the number of T cells and antibodies can cause the immune system to overreact so that the body begins to attack its own tissues. An example of this is rheumatoid arthritis.

On a more positive note, it was found that meaningful social contact increased the body's immune response. A satisfying marriage or the presence of even one meaningful relationship in one's life, was shown to be important in maintaining a high level of T cell functioning. When nursing home patients were given just one plant to care for, they became more alert, active, and interested in life.

This has been just a brief synopsis of the scientific facts. There will be more evidence in the coming years that will show that this mind/body link is strong, maybe stronger than we thought, perhaps stronger than we can even imagine. There are several books which illustrate and reference in detail the scientific evidence of the mind/body connection. Dr. Joan Borysenko is a scientist who's research spans from cell biology of Cancer to the state of the art in the medical sciences, called psychoneuroimmunology. Basically what this field does is bridge the gap between many of the fields of science to study the effects of our thoughts and mental state on the chemistry of the nervous system, which in turn affects the chemistry and functioning of our immune system. She explains this well, and in practical terms in her book, Minding the Body, Mending the Mind.

Dr. Bernard Siegel takes us through many accounts of exceptional patients in his books. He draws in scientific, philosophical, and psychological material from a variety of sources, forming a mosaic in this intertwining of the mind and the body, His illustrations are real people. This material is well referenced in the Notes Section of his book Peace, Love, and Healing, and is scattered throughout his book Love, Medicine, and Miracles.

One of the first persons to study the effect of induced relaxation on the physiology of the body, was a cardiologist at Harvard Medical School by the name of Dr. Herbert Benson. His book, The Relaxation Response, has become a classic. In it, he presents his research which addresses the **physiological** changes which occur in the body as a result of practicing meditation, where the body sustains a level of deep rest. All of his writing addresses the mind/body connection. One of his books that I highly recommend is, Your Maximum Mind.

So what does all of this mean to you practically? And how can you use this connection to your advantage so that you can become painfree and get on with your life? Before we can answer this fully we must take a look at the flip side of this connection, which is whatever happens to the body also has an effect on the mind. Every event that happens to you, every experience that you have, affects your mental/emotional self. A ride on a roller coaster elicits feelings of high adventure for some and feelings of fear for another. These feelings are unique to you.

When you are out walking on a beach in the evening and a cool breeze begins to blow upon your skin you may start to feel cool. And that feeling as the goosebumps begin to form may be pleasant or uncomfortable. So what starts as a physical event, the wind blowing, elicits an emotional response, discomfort or pleasure.

You see, we cannot experience anything without our thoughts and feelings joining the experience. The two become one. The experience cannot be separated from your feelings about the experience.

This jaw problem is an event in your life which you have lots of thoughts and feelings about. These thoughts and feelings are part of your physical pain. Often they resolve when the physical pain begins to resolve. But it is possible that your feelings can lead to an inner conflict which can impede the progress of therapy. You can be receiving the finest care available, but if you continue to harbor anger toward the driver of the car that hit you, or blame your spouse for causing your pain, you will continue to clench your jaw and have pain.

Occasionally psychotherapy may be necessary if these patterns are deeply seated. But more often what I see as necessary, is a willingness to be open to examining some areas of conflict in the life, and then taking some steps to change this for the better. When this work is begun, invariably the pain also begins to resolve.

Again, we are not talking here about Freudian analysis, critiquing your toilet training or early suckling habits. We are talking about identifying and releasing underlying thoughts and feelings about your pain or how you perceive how you got your pain. The effort you put into becoming aware of these factors for yourself will be time well spent and will enhance the effects of therapy. It may not always be an emotional conflict which is hindering the therapy, but when it is, it needs to be released on this level so that progress on a physical level can be resumed.

This is all that I am going to say about this very important aspect of your healing process. A lot of good books have been written on improving your lot by removing your emotional road blocks. I would greatly encourage those interested in pursuing this area of self discovery, for it is greatly life enhancing. Some favorite authors that I have found along the way are, Dr. Scott Peck, Dr. Wayne Dyer, and Dr. Judith Viorst. Some of their books are listed in the bibliography. There are countless others whose words inspire and challenge us to go farther, and dig deeper, to become more than we are and all that is possible.

MAKING THE CONNECTION

Creative Visualization

Sales of Harlequin romance novels are at a record high because wonderful bodily sensations can be awakened by the mental pictures we form while reading a book. Movies serve a similar purpose. A movie can be enormously pleasurable for the senses, the popcorn for the taste buds, and the sights and sounds which transport us into another time and place.

In many ways the body cannot tell the difference between the actual event or a mental picture of it. The body reacts similarly in terms of its internal functioning whether it is imagining, dreaming, or actually experiencing. We can use this phenomenon to our advantage. This is called creative visualization and you do it every time you read a book, go to the movies, or have a day dream. The only difference is that you can learn to direct it to help you put into your life what you most want.

When I first suggest to patients that they can use their thoughts to influence their pain many people invariably think that I think that their problem is in their head. I do not think that their problem is in their head. What I do think is that many people miss the obvious, which is that they can use the creative potential of the mind to help restore a painfree body.

Your mind puts into motion what you hold in it. Visualizing a healthy body in your mind can self propel the body into creating it. The success that you experience in your work can be linked to the creative efforts that you put forth in that direction. Yet, many do not see the connection with regards to the continued enjoyment of good health. A healthy body is often taken for granted. You may need to devote some time and energy in restoring some of the vitality that may be lacking. I hope that you will not see this as a burden but as an area of your life that needs some special attention. And do I dare suggest it could even be fun?

Do you remember at all what it felt like to be a child? Observing children can reeducate us to the wonderful world of play. Remember how we used to play all day, come into the house exhausted, fall into bed and sleep through until morning? I remember long summer days of playing with the neighborhood gang. When we were together we were never bored. We invented things. There was this empty lot next to our houses which we sort of took over. We guarded that field with our lives and really believed that it belonged to us. And in a way it did. We played our little hearts out in that field. And when I remember it I picture all of our faces and I think of innocence, fun, and adventure.

In using creative visualization you can capture that playful feeling that you had when you were a child. This could take many forms including silliness and nonsense. I hope these two things aren't entirely gone from your life. A little silliness can be very renewing. However, I must admit that sometimes you need to be discreet in these behaviors. For example, when certain people come to the house to visit I do hide the rubber duck and battery operated whale that sit on top of the bath tub. I don't have to do that very often though, since most of my friends are of the playful variety. Anyway, back to the discussion.

Being creative in seeing yourself achieve what you would like yourself to be or do can be fun as well as satisfying. And the more detail you can visualize around your goal the better. For example, let's say that your goal is to be able to return to your job as an interior designer in six months. You can picture yourself in someone's new home fully desgined by you. You can be sitting in your favorite room in the house, wearing a dress or T-shirt with the date stamped on it (six months from now). You can be smiling, radiant, and most of all, painfree. The mind loves pictures. Now it can create this one.

Another helpful exercise is to draw your pain on a piece of paper using colored chalk or pencils. Although this can be intimidating at first, it can be enlightening to see what the pain looks like on a piece of paper. This exercise also helps gets the pain out of you and onto the paper.

Let's say that you draw your pain as a rope. You can then give it qualities such as thick, steel-like, or constricting. You can color it and see what that color means to you. And now for the most important part, you can change it. The choice is yours. If cutting it is too direct for you, fray it, set it on fire, transform it into a balloon and have it float away. The possibilities are endless.

There are so many ways of enhancing the therapy using visualiz-ation. For example, your splint can become a magic tool working for you to put your jaw in the exact place it needs to be. If "magic" seems too far fetched for you make it something else that is mean-ingful for you. Many of my patients tell me that they hate their splints. I try to help them get out of that mind set immediately.

Hating something can negate the positive effects, no matter how right it may seem. Get the splint modified, adjusted, or change your thinking. If it is truly necessary for you to wear it, make it a useful support for your life.

Another way in which you can gain from this practice is to visualize the effects of the therapy creatively. For example, feel the heat from the hot pack treatment melting the **muscle spasm** away. See the muscles elongating and relaxing. Visualize what heat energy looks like coming off the pavement on a hot summer day, and feel it penetrate through your body in that same wavelike fashion. Native American Indians claim to draw strength from the bear, vision from the eagle, and gentleness from the deer. So why not draw healing energy from the hot pack?

If some of this seems silly to you, you are not alone. Many people have some initial inertia in beginning this practice. But what I can tell you is that once you start imagining more and playing with this, literally, it becomes easier to do and adds a whole new dimension to life. It also works, and the sky is the limit as to what you can accomplish. Creative visualization perhaps cannot solve all of your problems but it can certainly put them in a better light and help you to become more positive. Negativity will make reaching your goal impossible.

There is a superb book on this subject by one of my favorite authors, Shakti Gawain. The book is called Creative Visualization. In it, she describes in detail how you can become adept at creating in your life what you first visualize in your mind. When you begin this practice it soon becomes second nature, and in a very short time you begin to start working with yourself instead of fighting yourself every step of the way. What a nice way to live!

The Eleventh Commandment

Society is in desperate need of an eleventh commandment. And I believe that if God had known then what we were going to do with the other ten that he would have made this the eleventh Himself. That commandment is, "Thou shalt be responsible for ones own thoughts, feelings, and actions." Maybe we cannot control all of the events that happen to us in our lives, but we can control how we react to them and what we do about them.

We may know this intellectually but emotionally the tendency is there to blame external events and people for our own pain and suffering. "He made me feel" still echoes across the land. And the simple truth is that no one can make us feel anything. We do the choosing ourselves. No exceptions! And while it is true that events and people's behavior can be less than uplifting, still, they cannot make us feel anything.

When you really begin to make this connection for yourself on an emotional level, you will have illuminated your life with the brightest light available. Every aspect of your life will change when you begin to act in your life instead of react. So kick the pebble and start the avalanche.

Some people will go their entire lives without connecting that what we first desire in our hearts, think with our minds, and fuel with our imagination and determination, makes what happens, happen. This seems so apparent. Still, many people drift without focus or direction, and then wonder why life isn't working out for them. It doesn't work out unless you plan, take action, and stay determined.

Until you own this physical problem, or circumstance that you are in and take full responsibility for it, you will probably go from health professional to health professional and never get the help you really need to heal the condition. Do not entrust this responsibility to anyone but yourself. From this position you can then draw in the people that will help you help yourself.

The feeling that you want this pain to just be gone or taken away is universal. And you probably feel that you haven't asked for this. And you may not want to deal with it. The list of possibilities is long. I don't know anyone who would welcome this kind of pain. And yet here you are in this predicament. What do you do?

The first step is to accept that it is your responsibility to change this situation with help. Lots of lip service is paid to the fact that health care is the individual's responsibility, and people continue to go to doctors and therapists expecting them to take the pain away. On an inner level, inside of you, in that quiet place, right now, decide that healing this problem is your primary priority. Decide that you will be well again. This step you must do on your own. No one can help you with this one. It is between you and yourself.

In the story, The Dark Crystal, the skexis, who were the bad guys, captured the pod people, who lived in the community, drained their life essence and drank it in order to gain eternal youth and vitality. But the emperor skexis soon learned that the effects from the potion were short lived and even backfired, making him older before his time. Youth and vitality are qualities of the spirit that come from within. No short cuts are possible to attain them. The healing potential lies within you. There is no shortcut. You can search externally for a long time but you won't find it. True, you will need some help. But also true, you will ultimately be the one who makes the inner shift to a healthier life.

In summary, your body is an intricately designed masterpiece. Your mind is the creative powerhouse for your life. Making the body/mind connection work for you in restoring your well being begins with you taking responsibility for your physical health as well as your mental health. You can help restore your body to health by first creating a healthy vibrant body in your mind. Whatever you set your mind to do, you can do.

Setting Goals

Once you have assumed responsibility for your situation you are ready for the next step, setting goals. My favorite poster is of a newborn chick having just popped out of its shell. The caption says, "Now what?" So that you don't stand around in your new responsible position saying "now what" for too long you need to set realistic goals.

When I ask my patients how I can help them, they invariably say, "I want to feel better." But I don't know what "feel better" means to you. You may not even know what "feel better" means to you. Without a more concrete goal you are in the same position as the chick in the poster, in transition, out of the egg but not into life. You've assumed responsibility but for what purpose?

So right now, on a piece of paper write down what you want, and what that would allow you to do. Complete this sentence. I want (to be) _____ so that I can (do) _____.

For example, let's say you want to be painfree so that you can get back to work full time and begin cooking dinners for your family again. "Feeling better" is now defined and you can begin visualizing yourself painfree at work and cooking in the kitchen. A goal of being painfree so that you can walk four miles three times per week is pretty clear. These are the kinds of goals that it is necessary for you to come up with. The goals must be meaningful to you or you won't want to work to achieve them.

Answers that are not acceptable are, "get back to my life," "be happier," "feel better," or anything that leaves room for interpretation. There is a big difference between getting better and being painfree. That difference is the same as thinking about something as opposed to doing it, or starting something as opposed to finishing it. A goal to become painfree for a purpose has more determination behind it than a goal to feel better. It suggests a deeper commitment to the process. And until one is committed there is a hesitancy which breeds failure. Moving onward in boldness one is more likely to achieve the goal that if one sets his sights below the mark.

So dare to state your plan to be painfree. And whatever it is that you want to be able to do, dare to get excited about it. Let your deepest desires surface. Use this as an opportunity to move ahead.

If you are finding goal setting difficult you are not alone. All of my patients find this part hard to do. Often I find myself having to pull this information out of people. But this part is critical to the therapy. I would like to elaborate on this a little further since it is so important.

So many doctors and therapists treat patients and never know what it is that the patient wants. This is hard to believe, but true. We have no idea what you want when you come through our doors. You need to be as clear as you possibly can as to what your needs are and what your end goal is. We will better know how to proceed in the therapy if we know what sorts of activities you need to be able to return to, and the general time frame you have in mind. We will also be able to advise you on how realistic those aspirations and time frames are. Our work with you then becomes purposeful and your efforts in the therapy become purposeful.

Achieving the Goal

Nothing happens without effort. And the biggest effort that you will have to put forth is the emotional effort of continuing on, even when the responsibility that you have accepted feels overwhelming, and when your goals seem cloudy, unreachable, and vague. This is when you need to pull in all of your reserves. There will be good professionals helping you and this is the time to air your doubts or get some bolstering. Call on your friends. Call on your faith. Find or do something uplifting. Whatever you do, don't stay in the doldrums.

Remaining in a state where you are continuously upset is a hindrance to your progress toward your goal. Use your emotion to your advantage, don't let your emotion use you. Use the energy that you are now using to complain or feel sorry for yourself to solve the problem. You are hurting yourself the most by harbouring and reinforcing these thoughts. Become aware if you are doing this. Redirect your thinking. Use the emotion, don't let it use you.

There are many things that you can do to keep yourself in a good place mentally. There is a wonderful little book called, What To Do When You're Feeling Blue, by Mark Schneider and Ellen Meyer. Find that little book! Read positive affirmations such as the Hazelton series, the Daily Word, or Bible passages. Listen to music. It can be a mood elevator. There is a variety of "anti-frantic" music on the market today, some accompanied by positive affirmation. Become absorbed in a good story book. Study a painting or photograph.

The most meaningful part of my life besides the love shared with family and friends is the fulfillment that I receive in my work. I have the priviledge of being able to help people transform their lives. I see people who come to me in great distress become productive and happy again. It is a great joy to see this happen. And what I notice about the people who achieve their goals versus the ones who don't is this; the people who make it, take and use all that I give, and demand the best of me. I can want it for you and do, but what really counts is that you want it for yourself. You have to take it from whatever source and use it for yourself.

A great teacher once told me that if you took what you knew and turned it completely around, that it would be closer to the truth. It would appear as if I, the therapist, am the teacher and you, the patient, the student. But perhaps you become the teacher for me, pointing the way, giving the direction. Each patient teaches me for the next and you should be zealous in your desire to teach your doctors and therapists.

I am not talking about spouting off technical information about your diagnosis. What I mean is telling what you know to be true for you right now about what is happening in your body. Help us. We need the help so that we can help you.

This situation that you find yourself in, this problem that you are in the middle of which may seem to you to be insurmountable can bring you through a series of experiences which can change your life forever if you will let it. You can learn from it. You can grow from it. You can become a better human being because of it.

Wisdom approaches slowly. You may not get immediate answers. But be ever watchful for its unfoldment. For in years to come you may look back and gain valuable insight from the unpleasant experience of today.

This pain is perhaps one the of most difficult hardships that you will have to overcome in your life. That is why it is so important to hold your goal in your awareness. Be prepared for setbacks, but walk as straight and narrow a path until it is achieved. Picture your proud achievement and make it happen.

IT WILL TAKE AS LONG AS IT TAKES

On a warm spring day in 1983 I went flying through the air off the back of my horse, twisting, tumbling, and awkwardly landing across the width of an olympic size arena. Had I kept tumbling I would have been all right. But my jeans got caught on the side wall of the arena abruptly halting my pelvis. The accident happened in slow motion. And when I stopped, the world seemed to stop too. The lumbar discs tore, the sacroiliac joint tore and the pelvis was badly compressed from the impact. It was a serious injury. And over the course of the next five years I was to learn what it was like to be a real patient.

The pain was excruciating. The doctors had little to offer since nothing was broken. My left leg was numb all of the time, and walking felt impossible. I could not go to the grocery stores or malls because the concrete floors would hurt my back. For over two years I ate what I could buy at the drive up Farm Store window. Work was a nightmare for the first year.

I was chiropractored. acupunctured, massaged, physical therapied, rolfed, and doctored. I went through a lot physically, emotionally, and spiritually and I would like to share with you what I learned.

The body heals in its own way in its own time, and it takes as long as it takes. This teaches patience but can lead to frustation, because it seems never fast enough. After two years I could turn in bed without pain and sleep through the night. After three years I could walk without pain but any extra effort would set me back months. In the fourth year I began to do more and feel less pain. Five years later the problem is well healed, but the area is vulnerable and needs attention often. I look back on my process with great wonder. A part of me marvels that it could heal at all. And I am grateful.

There is an interesting phenomenon about pain that I learned. When you hurt, you can't remember what it feels like to feel good. And when you feel good, you can't remember what it feels like to hurt. I used to have three good days, feel some pain on the fourth and claim I never felt good. On the other hand when I had a day without pain I could not remember what the pain was like. This aspect of pain is so curious to me. Many of my patients report the same.

Another way in which this presents itself is that as patients start to get better they don't remember how bad they were in the beginning. Even though the pain may still be present at times, it is nowhere near the severity. It is just that they don't remember.

Another phenomenon about pain is that on a day when your mood is somewhat depressed, it is hard to tell if the pain is actually worse or if you just don't feel as good that day. For me, there was a strong connection here so I worked doubly hard to stay above it mentally. What I noticed was that when I would be a little down in the morning, the pain would be more apparent, which would depress me a little more, which would increase the pain. So staying as positive as I could, although it took effort, helped me keep my pain under control.

And I learned other things. This experience taught me to slow down, to pace myself. It took a little wind out of my hell-bent attitude to prove something. I don't take the ability to move freely, easily, and painfree for granted anymore. I enjoy the way my body feels when I hike in the woods or ride my bicycle through the village where I live. And I have gained a valuable insight about my life.

During my formative years I developed this large chip on my shoulder. When I would get pretty high and mighty, my very big, very strong father would grab my wrist hard, which would paralyze me emotionally as well as physically. He would grit his teeth, look me in the eye and say, "Get down off your high horse, kid." I would look at my wrist for the black and blue marks but there never were any. Anyway, that would keep me humble for a good six months before he had to do it again.

After my dad died that great check on my life, to keep me on track, was gone. I believe on one level that I created that experience of falling off my high horse, to be a constant reminder for the rest of my life that I am no better that anyone else. So when I feel a little twinge from time to time I am reminded of my place in humanity alongside everyone else who is trying to make it just like me.

We have a get rid of it attitude in this culture. if we don't like something, or something is uncomfortable we dispose of it. But I tell you that what you must do is go into the pain to get through it. If you ignore it or push it aside it will just show up in another way in your life. Pay attention to your pain. Learn its lessons well. Let it soften you to life. Let it take as long as it takes.

CONCLUSION

The inner you is vast uncharted territory. In the course of reading this chapter, I hope that you have grown somewhat familiar with the territories within you that can lead you back to physical wholeness.

In Columbus's time, there were people who believed that the earth was flat, and people who believed that the earth was round. And to those standing on the dock it appeared as if the boat, as it reached the horizon, fell off the end of the earth. But for those travellers who lost sight of lands just left, new shores came into view. The horizons of their minds widened at the same time their perspective of the earth changed. So step onto your ship and go to the helm. Release the ropes that hold you to the dock and sail in quest of your inner vision.

And for the times that you want to turn your ship around, here is some wonderful advice from my friend, Kate. Kate says that sometimes you just need to pull over on the side of the road (of life), and have a fresh peanut butter and jelly sandwich. It is sometimes the little things in life, the simple pleasures, that help us to reconnect with ourselves, like a peanut butter and jelly sandwich. So, have as many as you need, or do what you need to do to keep connected with yourself and keep yourself on course.

For many, a long time ago, the earth was flat. But for a few, their truth was that the earth was round. Today, many would have you believe that pain is a part of life and that you have to learn to live with it. But the greater truth is that in every living thing is a spirit longing to be free; free from limitation, free from lack, and free from pain.

I salute my fellow journeymen and feel a connectedness with all of you whether you are at full sail or at the dock eating a peanut butter and jelly sandwich. For we know that the living spirit is greater and more enduring that anything which tries to oppose it.

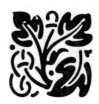

Patient
Stories

hen I say "I", I mean a thing
absolutely unique, not to be confused
with any other.

— Ugo Betti

ix

This chapter has been written by my patients. The stories that they tell about their experiences with TMJ and headache have been unedited, except for punctuation and grammar. These stories speak for themselves.

I am a 37 year old housewife. I can remember getting headaches as early as age 7. I continued getting them periodically through the years.

After my son was born, when I was 25, I would get monthly headaches that would last a few days. I was on birth control pills at the time. When I was pregnant with my second child, I never had a headache during the entire pregnancy (which made me think they were hormonally related). After my daughter was born the headaches returned, but much more severely. I was then advised by my doctor to discontinue the use of the birth control pills, but the headaches still continued.

Finally, after an eight day headache, I decided to see my family doctor. He ordered an EEG (electroencephelogram), which was normal, and prescribed various medications, which did not help. The pain would begin above my right eye, and the right side of my head, face, and neck would hurt. The headaches would normally last from two days to one week. I would end up in bed unable to stand noise, food, or light, and be unable to think straight. Once the headaches subsided, I felt weak, depressed, and washed out.

I found it increasingly difficult to care for my babies. There were times when my husband had to come home from work to take care of the children.

I started seeing a chiropractor thinking that if I could get some of my neck and back pain relieved that it would help relieve my headaches. I saw her for two years. But my headaches were getting more and more severe. I was getting them more often and they would last longer.

I then started seeing a neurologist, and he diagnosed migraine headaches. I remember that my mother got migraine headaches until menopause, and I remember thinking that I couldn't wait that long to stop having these headaches. So I started taking a variety of drugs (beta blockers etc.). Nothing seemed to keep them from coming and the only thing that made them go away was Cafergot.

It started to become a vicious cycle. After I got rid of one with the Cafergot, I would go to bed and wake up with yet another headache. Just when I thought they could not get worse I would develop one that would last eight days. I found that I could not eat or sleep, and I had taken all of the Cafergot I could take.

When all else failed the doctor admitted me to the hospital. I was almost relieved because I thought at last I would get some answers.

I had extensive testing, which consisted of another EEG, CT scan, and blood work, only to find out they were just migraines, and I had to learn to live with them. They told me that I may get relief when I go through menopause, and to take drugs indefinitely.

The headaches were interfering with every aspect of my life. I was afraid to go on vacation or plan ahead for entertaining. I felt guilty because I was unreliable. I had to cancel plans all the time because of how I felt. I became resentful of people telling me to relax and suggesting to me that I had a "migraine personality." I was determined to find someone that could help me!

A friend of mine called me one day and told me of this doctor in Erie, Pa., that did cranial therapy for headache sufferers. I felt I had nothing to lose.

The first thing he told me was that I was not crazy. And he said he could help me. In addition to the cranial therapy he referred me to a dentist who diagnosed TMJ. They had me follow a special diet which consisted of no dairy products, limited caffeine, white sugar, and wine. I was also instructed to go off all drugs, except Cafergot when I got a headache.

I was fitted for an appliance (splint) that I wore day and night. I could remove it during eating. I was told that once my jaw became stable that I would need braces. I continued to see this doctor for about 1 year and was 80% better. I still continued to get headaches around my menstrual cycle. At that time I was also told to see a physical therapist. That's when I think I started to see real improvement.

I was doing very well, but periodically I would have a relapse. Once again I would get discouraged and depressed but I continued with the therapy.

I was then told by the doctors in Erie, Pa. about a physical therapist in Philadelphia who used myofascial release techniques. I talked it over with my husband and we decided that I should go for treatment. I thought maybe I needed to go just one more step before getting well. It was quite a commitment because it meant leaving my family for a week. I ended up making the trip three times. I call it a commitment because when you decide to see a therapist it usually takes patience and time to undo all of the damage. It does not get better overnight.

My emotions have been like a roller coaster. Every time I seek help, I hope that this is the answer, and that I will never get another headache.

On my last trip to Philadelphia I felt very upset at times. I kept thinking that if this treatment did not work, I wouldn't know where else to go. So far I really feel this treatment along with my weekly sessions with my therapist has helped me.

I feel many things contributed to my headaches, my menstrual cycle, my diet, my misaligned body, and my TMJ. It is so difficult to figure out because it isn't any one thing. So far now, I am off drugs, and I am on hold with my jaw. I continue to receive therapy weekly.

I feel that the quality of my life has truly changed for the better since I've gotten relief from my headaches. I am happier. I feel that I look better. I feel like I can plan for the future. I feel like a better wife and mother. I also feel very fortunate to have found the people who helped me.

Over a year ago, in the course of what I thought was to be a totally normal day, began the most horrible time of my 35 years of existence. I worked until 4:00 and picked up my kids to run some errands. We stopped at the local Burger King for supper, and went to the laundromat to wash clothes. On the way home, we were broadsided by an out-of-control car. My car spun around 90 degrees, jumped a curb, and was stopped by a telephone guide wire. Apparently, according to my children, I just sat there for some time and moaned. My younger boy kept shaking me, and calling me until I answered. I don't know how long I sat there. I wandered around the parking lot in total confusion, only intermittently remembering things, while the police did their thing. The boys were quite shaken, but in a couple of days they were feeling back to normal. I still don't know if I was knocked unconscious, or hit my head or face on anything in the car.

I saw my doctor the next day. I could not walk upright, and I could barely move my neck. I could not lift my arms, talk, or get in or out of a chair. TALK ABOUT MUSCLE SPASMS! For the first month I took muscle relaxants, antidepressants, anti-inflammatories, and eventually tranquilizers. My best friends were my moist heating pad and a hot bath. I could not even do simple household chores. I could not stand, lay, or sit in the same position for more than 15 minutes at a time. I got dizzy if I sat or stood too long. I had blurred vision (intermittently) for about 3 months. I still get into a weird, confused, vague state of mind sometimes. When I feel like this, I can't concentrate on even the simplest, routine matters.

These symptoms made me feel and think that I was going crazy, or having a nervous breakdown. My family thought this too. At times I would become totatly irrational, and get out of control emotionally over really nothing. My doctor gave me a mild tranquilizer which did help. Through the assurance and comforting from my doctors and physical therapist, I was convinced that I was not going nuts. As my treatments continued and the pain began to subside, I began to feel better emotionally as well as physically.

One month after the accident, my doctor sent me to a physical therapist. Here I lucked out. She discovered my TMJ problem. I told her all my problems which included restriction in opening my mouth, as well as snapping and pain, which was really bad when I opened my mouth. Here we go, my adventure with TMJ Syndrome! This is a medical term for physical, emotional, psychological, and spiritual pain!

Nothing aggravated me more than having one of the medical professionals ask, "How are your headaches?" This simple question still makes my skin crawl. Let me tell you what a TMJ headache is like, and I have since found out that this is typical. Pain totally engulfs your head, inside and out, your face, teeth, ears, neck, under your lower jaw, and even cervical spine area. Pain usually starts at the base of my skull and shoots up the back of my head, comes around the sides and under my ears, up the sides of my face (the inside of my ears really hurt now), and into my temples. Now you tell me, is this a headache? No, this is head pain.

This has affected my sex life tremendously, stressed all of my relationships and affected how I feel about myself. Between the physical, mental/emotional trauma that sets in, and then the people around you questioning whether you're putting on or not, depression sets in. This is where my doctors and physical therapist really helped me. Because they were seeing me regularly, they observed how one day I seemed good, and the next I was in terrible shape. They called each other and discussed my condition. I knew they really cared about me. My dentist would even call me at home to see if I was feeling better. If you're as lucky as I am you will find these kinds of caring medical people.

I did have an arthrogram of the left jaw. It showed that I have a dislocated disc in my jaw. The ligaments that control disc movement are damaged. The medical diagnosis is pretty much dislocated jaw and torn/damaged surrounding soft tissue. But my neck and jaw injuries are so closely related that when one acts up, so does the other.

My dentist and physical therapist have coordinated splint therapy and physical therapy to realign my jaw. This is a very slow, hard process. I have good days, and I have bad days. I am learning true patience. So far, so good. They're trying to keep me out of surgery and it looks like that's how it will be.

I thank God for my husband's help and support, and also my boys. I don't know what I would have done without them. I still have to count on them to do things I can't do. I am back to work after seven months off, working full time in an office.

Whatever you do, don't let anyone make you think the problem is made up, or blown out of proportion. Looking at you from the outside, they can't always tell what you're going through on the inside. Have someone you can talk to, preferably more than one.

Find a good understanding doctor, that knows about TMJ, or at least is willing to learn (mine has learned a lot from my case). Do what you are told. At least try. Give it a chance. With TMJ there is no fast cure. Oh yeah, find a good lawyer who has had experience with TMJ cases. You will quickly find out that insurance companies do not want to pay for TMJ Syndrome. They will claim that it is not from the accident. They call it a preexisting condition.

I have a helpful hint for my fellow sufferers. If the muscles on the inside of your mouth by the back of your teeth hurt, buy a slurpee, slushee, slush drink (I don't know what it is called in your area). It is slushed ice flavored with syrup. Sip it and let it melt in the area that hurts. It will numb that area and give you relief. It's colder that milk shakes or ice cream and you won't be choking on ice chips.

I know my case is not the worst case. I read anything I could find on TMJ. It was comforting for me to know that I was not the only one with this. The only reason I wrote this was to share some of the problems I have gone through in the hope it may help someone else.

God Bless.

I am a forty five year old woman who is a homemaker. I'm finding it a little difficult remembering just when my headaches began. I guess they started when I was a child of about ten or twelve years old. I was shy and I think that's when I started keeping a lot of feelings to myself. I also had a couple of injuries. Once I banged my jaw on the bath tub. Another time I got hit in the forhead with a baseball bat. I don't know if these incidents had any bearing on my headaches. In those days you didn't run to the doctor for every little accident. We just couldn't afford it financially. When I compare the headaches that I got then to the ones I get now, the ones I got in the past don't seem too bad. My headaches have gotten worse over the years.

When I was sixteen, my mother took me to a chiropractor. I went for a couple of treatments. I hated the feeling of my bones being cracked, so I decided not to go back. Ever since the treatments, my bones are always cracking. I am really sorry I ever went in the first place.

It was shortly after my first daughter was born that I went to a neurologist. He sent me for brainwave studies and X-rays which were negative. The diagnosis was tension headaches. He put me on tranquilizers which made me tired all of the time. So I stopped taking them, and just relied on pain killers.

Several years later I was hospitalized for dizziness. I had more brainwave studies, more X-rays, and also a CT scan. All were negative. It turned out to be a problem with my inner ear.

Not a day would go by without me taking some kind of pain killer. So many of the prescription drugs did not agree with me, so I just took Anacin 3 for a lot of years. It was just a temporary relief, not a cure. I worried about what all those pills were doing to me, but I didn't know what else to do.

I used to pray that they would find something wrong with me, so that they could correct it. Most days my headaches consist of a tightness in my head, which I can tolerate with medication. Then there's what I call my bad headaches. It's a constant throbbing on one side of my temple and up the back of my head. My pain medication doesn't help. All I can do is lie down with ice pack after ice pack. Sometimes they last for a couple of days. I do a lot of praying at those times.

I don't think most people can understand what its like to have these constant headaches. They can sympathize with you, but unless you experience the constant pain, you can't realize the effect it has on that person. Sometimes it hurts when relatives make a joke about it. They jokingly have said, "Oh, you can't plan on her, she'll probably have one of her famous headaches," or that its all in her head and laugh.

My husband and children are great. I get a lot of consideration from all of them. But again, I don't think they can really understand the toll it takes on me. At times I feel very depressed and think, why me? But then I think of all of the people that are worse off than I am, and it helps me cope.

I also feel very guilty about all of the special occasions that were spoiled because of me. I almost hate to plan anything. I think I try so hard not to have one of my bad headaches that I actually cause myself to have one. Just this past year, my Thanksgiving and Christmas were spoiled by my headaches.

I first became aware of TMJ when I read an article in a magazine about headaches. I read another article in the newspaper. The article was about a research program at the University of Buffalo, which dealt with headaches being caused by jaw problems. The people mentioned in the article sounded like me. They reported having headaches every day, constantly taking pills, never getting any relief. I should have called UB then. Instead, I looked in the phone book for a dentist who might specialize in TMJ. I found one and went to see her. She sounded like she could help me. She took X- rays of my jaw, and measured me for a splint. I had to wear the spint all of the time. I would go once a week to get an adjustment on the splint. The adjustment took two minutes. The visit cost twenty-six dollars. After over six months and over a thousand dollars I stopped treatment, because I wasn't getting anywhere.

I had kept the newspaper article about the TMJ program at the University. I didn't know just how to go about it so I just called UB, and they set up an appointment for an evaluation of my problem.

I was accepted into their program. The charge was minimal compared to my dental cost. Everyone I met was so understanding and kind, especially the doctor that was assigned to me.

I began biofeedback training to learn to relax my jaw and neck muscles. I went once a week. I started listening to my relaxation tape every day. I had some jaw exercises to do. And I kept a pain diary between visits.

My headaches are getting better. I very seldom clench my teeth anymore. I'm taking much less medication. I do have a constant stiffness in my neck and pain in the back of my head. So my doctor recommended a physical therapist for me to see.

I've started physical therapy. I have high hopes that maybe this will be my final answer. My muscles are very tight and need to be relaxed. I feel really good after each treatment, but I think it will probably take a while for me to say I feel really good. But I feel it is going to happen.

I find it hard to believe none of my doctors ever suggested to me that it could be a jaw problem. My knowledge came from reading magazine and newspaper articles. I never realized how many people have a problem with headaches until recently. I agreed to write this story for this book because it may help someone else with the same problem who doesn't know where else to turn.

I am a religious person. I feel my prayers and the Novenas my husband and I make, finally steered me in the right direction. I thank God that there are people who care enough about other people's pain, who work to help alleviate it, so that we can lead a more full and happier life.

I am a 34 year old woman who has a family. In addition, I have worked, and consider myself a good homemaker. I have had headaches for many years. My dentist made a splint, and it worked well for nine months. Then I had a car accident, which sprained my neck, and aggravated my TMJ. The dentist began treating me again, and called in the neurologist, who referred me to physical therapy. The therapy increased my muscle spasms and made me feel worse. I was then referred to the Erie County Medical Center because the neurologist was puzzled. At this point the pain was so bad I had no strength in my arms or hands, and I couldn't turn my neck normally.

The Medical Center confirmed that it was a sprained neck and TMJ and prescribed drug therapy. Then I was referred to the University of Buffalo TMJ Clinic.

Aside from me not being able to move my arms well, or move my neck from side to side or turn it, my ear was numb, and my neck and shoulders were in such spasm, they felt like they were burning. The doctors at the University could hardly examine me, I was in such bad shape. Also I had two abscessed teeth, but couldn't get root canals done because I couldn't open my mouth.

I began biofeedback and a mild muscle relaxant. Within six months I was able to have the root canal. Also, I began to decrease considerably my pain medication (which I was taking every 2 hours).

After about a year of biofeedback, my doctor suggested that I receive physical therapy. I've received two months of therapy and am feeling a lot better. My therapist has done more for me in the last few months than anybody. I feel that I will be completely well. It has been 20 months since my accident. Even though the doctors told me I would never be cured, I know I will.

I truly do not think anyone can comprehend the pain and the emotions I was going through, unless they have been through it. I wasn't able to do anything because the pain was so bad. And when I felt a little better and did things, it would put me to bed.

I would get very frustrated because my house was a mess. My family would help clean, but I felt useless. The girls tried to understand, but they got sick of hearing," Mommy can't because she doesn't feel good." I would be very miserable, and at times would take it out on my family. I couldn't stand the pain.

Our whole lives were drastically changed. Before my accident I worked full time, and was very involved with my family. After the accident I remember cheering my daughter on in a swim meet, and going into severe spasm. Because I couldn't work, our budget got very tight, which upset me.

I gained a lot of weight, and was very depressed. My parents and sister enrolled me into a diet program, and I lost the weight, which makes me feel better about myself. I would fight with my husband because I would think he didn't understand. He did, but I didn't think he knew all of the emotions and pain I was going through.

The one thing that kept me going was fighting the pain. I refused to stay that way. I am a very stubborn person. I had a will to get better and get on with my life.

Today, I still have pain, but it is nothing like it was. I am getting more energy, and doing more things. Sometimes I get more pain when I overdo, but at least I am not back in bed. I went on my first vacation, and walked the entire Magic Kingdom at Disney World. My family kept offering to get me a wheelchair, but I didn't need it. That felt really good.

I am a 33 year old woman who supports myself, and has a very active lifestyle. My experience with TMJ has plagued me for the past three and a half years. The trauma it has caused me, comes into perspective as being both physical and emotional, the physical, being dull to agonizing pain in my right jaw, ear, neck, and shoulder, and the emotional stemming from the almost constant pain due to the unanswered questions and unsuccessful treatments. My outlook on TMJ is very bleak. I almost want to inform people with this condition to do nothing, although when you're in so much discomfort you will seek any type of help. I feel justified in making that statement, since I feel I have made enough attempts to get diagnosed and cured with this ailment. I will explain my case.

My first attack of TMJ occurred with my bite misaligning. Out of nowhere, my jaw changed its position. It lasted for a couple of days, and then adjusted itself back to normal, or so it seemed. Unfortunately, after that incident, I became more aware of a cracking and grinding noise in the joint upon opening. No pain was prominent yet, but I did decide to see my dentist. The dentist determined that the jaw bone did slip out of position in the socket. He made a bite plate that covered my upper teeth, that I wore at night. This was to help reposition the bone, and prevent clenching or grinding of my teeth.

I wore the plate for a couple of months, when other symptoms started to occur. I started getting bad headaches associated with tunnel vision. Never thinking that this was connected with the jaw, I went to see an optician and then an opthamologist. Both examined my eyes thoroughly and found nothing to be wrong. However, they did suggest that I see a neurologist because the incident happened more than once.

Within a seven month period, I started experiencing a burning pain in the back of my right ear, down the neck and into the shoulder. The headaches were also continuing. I went to see the neurologist. I went through a neurological exam, a CT scan, and had cervical X-rays taken. I was diagnosed with migraine headaches. The treatment consisted of medication and the elimination of certain irritants. That method helped the head pain a little, but the burning pain was almost constant now. The neurologist referred me to an ear, nose, and throat doctor to rule out an ear or sinus problem, and to check the small lump that I had behind my ear.

I arrived at the ENT doctor's office hoping for an answer. He diagnosed the lump to be a harmless nodule, my sinuses to be chronic, and my jaw to be completely off in its alignment. He felt the jaw was causing most of the burning pain. He explained that the muscles around the jaw joint were in spasm, causing my bite to shift. He prescribed muscle relaxants, and recommended that I see a dentist specializing in TMJ. I finally was mentally relieved that this ENT doctor knew what was causing the pain.

After two months of taking muscle relaxants, I went to the TMJ dentist. I felt the relaxants were not helping enough because my jaw would lock shut at times. The dentist assembled an extra piece of plastic on my original bite plate, so that my back teeth did not make contact upon closing. That was supposed to relieve the muscles around the jaw. After wearing the plate for a few months I began to sense that this treatment was not working. The pain down my neck and shoulders would still get intense. Medication was not helping. At that point I decided to stop this method, and hope for the best.

It was fifteen months since the start of this nightmare that the pain just got unbearable. I did not know where to go or who to see for help. Finally, I heard from a friend, about a physical therapist who dealt with TMJ. I called her immediately and was evaluated. She replied that she could help, using hot packs and deep muscle massage. I knew after the first therapy session that this treatment was the answer. As she worked on the muscles of my neck and shoulder, I would feel the pain into my jaw and head. I never suspected that those muscles had any connection with the jaw area. By relieving the muscle spasms, a lot of my burning intense pain and headaches were gone. It took a few months before the pain became very minimal. I still kept up the sessions once or twice a month for the next two years. The jaw would still pop and crack, but at least the agonizing pain vanished.

The therapist and I both knew that we were keeping the pain under control. Eventually the jaw would need more attention. So I sought out another dentist specializing in TMJ. This doctor found that the jaw bone was not centered in the jaw socket, where it normally should be resting. In other words, it slipped off the disc, and was pushing into the ear zone. That was supposedly why I was dizzy at times, and why the cracking and grinding noise was present upon opening. So his intention was to realign the jaw, by having me wear this different bite plate. This plate held my lower jaw forward, to get the bone back properly on the disc. I was to eat and sleep with it in place, 24 hours a day, for two to eight months. It was very difficult to get used to but I felt I must try this procedure because the jaw itself was not getting better.

Upon wearing the plate for three weeks, I did have some relief. The dizziness was gone, along with the cracking and grinding noise. In spite of that, within seven weeks, other complications arose. From changing the jaw position I had extreme pressure in my head that lasted one week. The earlier burning pain in the back of the ear, moved to the front of the ear, down the jawline and into the ear. Also, my right arm weakened. In general, I thought I was going to go out of my mind. But after attending a few extra physical therapy sessions, most of these complications subsided, except for the jawline and ear pain. From reading the X-rays, the doctor as well as the physical therapist, felt that the jaw was in the correct position. The only logical consideration for the ear and jawline pain was the possibility that the realignment was a shock to my jaw, and that I needed more time to adjust.

I did pursue that logic for five months, until I just couldn't take the pain any longer. After talking it over with my therapist, I had the dentist readjust by bite plate to allow the jaw to go back, toward its original position. That did lessen the pain, but not enough. I then decided to start taking the plate out for a couple of minutes during the day. By doing so, it seemed to relieve the pain. I still had to eat with the plate in, but the dentist agreed with me to start taking it out an hour a day, to give the joint freedom of movement. Within two and one half months, the pain lessened considerably. The disc seemed to be in the right position, because the cracking noise was gone. All in all my whole body, and disposition felt better. I finally felt that the hell of this ordeal was seeing some light.

My next step was getting a consultation from the orthodontist. I was told that braces would most likely be needed to align the teeth for a proper bite, and to stabilize the jaw in the new position. Two out of three orthodontists just about refused to do any treatment, because I was still experiencing some pain. The third wanted an arthrogram done on the right side, to see if maybe the disc was torn, or still misaligned. In my personal opinion, the arthrogram should have been done before any realigning was done with bite plates. In my case though, the test showed that the disc was not torn, and it was in the proper position. But the left side appeared to have an abnormality in the closed position. The only way to check that out, was to have another arthrogram on the other side, which I refused to have done. It would have been too emotionally draining for me. It was not physically painful, but more mentally, because the doctor injects a needle with dye into the joint, while you open and close your mouth.

Because of what the arthrogram showed, the orthodontist said that he could not guarantee that wearing braces would relieve the pain. It was a chance I could take. I decided against it, and hoped that my teeth would meet again in a more normal bite.

It took six months for my bite to go back so that I could chew properly again. It does not crack anymore, and the pain is minimal. That, I attribute, to physical therapy. I believe that keeping the muscles in my jaw, neck, and shoulders pliable, lead to the pain subsiding. I still get a little burning and aching around my ear now and then, but it is nothing compared with when I wore the plate, or before this whole ordeal began.

In conclusion, I guess you could say that the plate did help reposition the disc. I also strongly believe that physical therapy treatments were the largest asset in relieving the majority of the pain. I just hope that the disc stability keeps me painfree in the years ahead. I do not want to go through the feelings of depression, anger, and hopelessness again. I hope that my case has not discouraged anyone from seeking professional help. If you feel you have TMJ, find a reputable specialist. Get different opinions before you have extensive work done. Make sure that the doctor works with physical therapists. I can almost guarantee that the therapy will relieve most of the agonizing pain, as it has in my case. As more research is being conducted, I trust that a positive cure is right around the corner for us sufferers. Hang in there and don't feel like you suffer alone.

I am a 50 year old woman whose focus in life is family. I've needed chiropractic adjustments for the past 22 years of my life, in order to have some sense of well being. I would have pain in my entire spine, down my legs, and all the way to the top of my head. Sometimes I would be dizzy. I went to my doctor and all the medical tests were negative. The chiropractor that I was seeing at the time thought that the TMJ might be involved, and sent me to a dentist who specializes in this area. The dentist began to adjust my jaw, using a splint, and I began to notice that I was getting some relief of pain throughout my body. At the same time, I had a new upper denture made, which opened up my bite more. This helped relieve a great deal of the pain for about a year. I required much fewer chiropractic adjustments.

The pain slowly began returning, and I had another splint made for my lower teeth. At the same time I was referred to physical therapy. I continued for one year. The treatments reduced a great deal of the pain. But what helped me the most was a tip she gave me about relaxing the jaw. If you put the tip of your tongue on the roof of the mouth, you can't clench your jaw. This was a tremendous help for me, since clenching my teeth had intensified my pain.

The other thing that I found very helpful, was the stretches she taught me for the whole body, the neck, and the jaw. Further, through her postive approach, she helped me regain my faith in myself, and instilled a confidence in me that I could get better.

I did well for a year, getting occasional chiropractic adjustments. Then I had another denture made, which was thicker and showed more gum, but I got used to the look quickly, because it made me feel so much better. I've had this new look, and feel for two years now.

I returned for another series of physical therapy treatments periodically over the next six months. I like to think of it as putting on the finishing touches. Going for treatment helped me put into perspective all of what I went through, and how it affected my life. It was a place where I could talk about what was happening to me. I have felt a psychological healing as well as a physical healing from the people who have helped me, as well as from my own effort.

Through my many years of pain and not knowing what was wrong, I was hurting on every level as a human being, physically, emotionally, and spiritually. I know now how important my mind is, through my thoughts, in keeping me well. Perhaps I had to live with the physical pain to gain some wisdom and knowledge. When I feel myself slipping mentally I try to remember to replace fear with faith and worry with hope. My prayer for one and all is that you too can find some wisdom in the experience, and pass it along to someone, like I have been able to do, so that another may be relieved of some of the suffering. Peace.

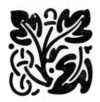

Endings

very seed bursts its container.
— Florida Scott-Maxwell

Seven

If you have made it to this point in the book, you are to be commended, for you have read through much information. As you become able to integrate this information, you will begin to gain an appreciation of the TMJ's simple complexity. In this final chapter, endings, we will summarize pertinent information from the various chapters, emphasize certain points, and draw some necessary conclusions. The first task will be to pull all of the information together in order to obtain some closure on the issues of TMJ and headache. We will review the common philosophies under which practitioners evaluate and treat TMJ and headache. We will emphasize the importance of musculoskeletal factors in relation to TMJ and headache. We will discuss the role that Western Medicine plays, as well as discuss alternative methods of treatment. And, we will once again touch on that inner private world of yours; that place where you process the events going on around you, that place which is you. So, let us begin our endings...

This book presents the basic, generic, stripped down, "uncola" version of TMJ **dysfunction** and headache. It is a solid account, based on common sense and sound treatment principles. The information presented is meant to enable you to sort through the conflicting material being presented by the media about TMJ and headaches, and offer some much needed hope. Even though controversy appears to abound regarding the cause, the solution is finally clear and simple: TMJ IS PRIMARILY A MUSCULOSKELE-

TAL PROBLEM. The anatomy of the TMJ is relatively the same as any other joint in the body. The inflammatory and healing processes are basically the same for all tissues. And the point of all of this is that we know how to treat joint problems very well. Just because the joint is anatomically situated in the head, only means that certain other factors need to be considered. These special considerations are primarily, the influence of the teeth on the functioning of the TMJ, and all of the medical implications due to the fact that the TMJ is so closely connected to the head anatomically.

So what appears to be so complex, and what has lead to so much confusion, in the end, becomes quite simple. TMJ is a problem with a joint and its surrounding structures. And when the basic treatment principles are applied to the TMJ, it heals and becomes pain free. You will remember those treatment principles to be, reduce pain, promote healing, restore range of motion, restore normal length and strength to the muscles, improve posture, reeducate the neuromuscular system through body awareness activities, and improve body mechanics to avoid further strain. So, my definitive comment on TMJ is that although it warrants certain other considerations, it is simply, a musculoskeletal condition amenable to treatment by methods which treat the musculoskeletal system.

When you seek help, be aware that your practitioner may belong to a particular "camp" whose members believe that TMJ has a specific cause, which warrants a specific treatment. For example, one "camp" believes that an imbalanced bite is the cause of TMJ. The tools that these practitioners use to remedy the situation are primarily **splint** therapy and reconstructive work in the mouth to change the bite. You will remember from an earlier discussion that some of these procedures are irreversible. Another "camp" is one of the behavioralists whose members believe that TMJ is caused by clenching and grinding behavior. The tools these practitioners use are **biofeedback** and/or drugs.

And then there is the "camp" to which I belong, which believes that muscle and its surrounding **fascia** is the primary cause of TMJ, and therefore the primary focus of treatment. The jaw, being dependent upon a balanced (mobile, straight, and strong) spine, functions only as well as the spine functions. The tools used by these practitioners, who are primarily physical therapists, were elaborated upon in the Physical Therapy Management Chapter. The members of this camp treat the muscles and joints directly, through a variety of techniques to restore the musculoskeletal system's resiliency.

In reality, several of these aspects may be operating to contribute to a person's condition. The schools of thought under which these "camps" operate, and the treatment modalities which they utilize are valid and effective in their own right. The critical question is who gets what, when? Let me give you a few examples to illustrate what I mean. If someone has a true mechanical problem, where the TMJ is locking, and they go to someone who believes in behavioral causes of TMJ, the person may be modifying their clenching behavior on a **biofeedback** machine, when what they really need is an **arthrogram** to detect a tear in the **disc** and surgery to repair it. If someone has a badly deteriorating set of teeth, resulting in a bite which is collapsing, you can establish the most perfect posture and reduce the **muscle spasms**, but what that person really needs is support from within the mouth for their TMJ. If someone has a forward head posture with considerable **muscle spasm** in the neck and facial areas, pulling the jaw forward mechanically by the use of a **splint** before the other factors are addressed will only add stress to an already overloaded system.

Having a broad view and good understanding of TMJ allows for many options to be exercised, so that a positive outcome can be achieved. Too narrow a view limits the treatment approach. You may have heard the saying that if all you have is a hammer, all you see is nails. All people are not nails, i.e. all people don't fall into one category. The truth is that TMJ has a variety of causes, and therefore a variety of treatment options are needed. The surgeons and dentists I work with are aware that any and all of these factors may be operating. And although we have to be in some "camp" and use some "hammer" in order to practice, we are not bound or limited by that. If someone is not responding to the treatment we administer, we know that another cause may be operating for that person and we send them on for consultation.

Now I would like to emphasize the importance of the musculoskeletal factors as they relate to TMJ. You will remember that we said eighty to perhaps ninety percent of all TMJ problems are muscular in origin. There are cases where the bite is a contributing factor. There can be mechanical problems within the joint itself. But most of the time TMJ is caused by a problem with muscle, often combined with joint tightness of the TMJ or the neck. Dr. Weldon

Bell, a dentist, has written extensively on orofacial pain, i.e. pain around the mouth and face areas. Dr. Bell states that almost all facial pain comes from the neck. Now why would a dentist make such a statement? He makes this statement because he knows that in a majority of cases it is not the teeth that are causing the problem, but rather, the muscles and joints in the surrounding areas, particularly the neck.

The neck is the base upon which the jaw functions, just as the trunk of a tree is the stable base from which the branches receive their support. Without the tree trunk the branches wouldn't branch, and without the neck the jaw wouldn't function. It is important that the neck be free of problems such as tightness or **muscle spasm**, because problems in the neck often cause problems in the jaw. You may remember the example from Chapter 4, of the **trigger point** in the anterior neck muscle referring pain into the face area. This is an example of how a problem in the neck can manifest itself in the TMJ area. Almost all of my TMJ patients and many of my headache patients have chronic neck complaints. THE IMPORTANCE OF FINDING AND SOLVING NECK PROBLEMS IS CRITCAL IN THE MANAGEMENT OF TMJ AND HEADACHE!

To further our discussion as to the importance of proper functioning of the musculoskeletal system in understanding and treating TMJ, good posture is a key ingredient. The TMJ is the last segment at the end of a long **kinetic chain** which begins with the feet coming in contact with the floor. Proper functioning of the whole spine, addressing the entire **kinetic chain** is important, and most necessary with regards to the neck. The jaw is sensitive to any change in the mechanics of any part of the body, from the feet, to the legs, through the entire spine. We have talked about forward head posture being the most common postural change that we observe in TMJ. As the head moves forward on the body, the jaw gets pulled back. This is only one example of how a change in the mechanics of one part of the body affects the TMJ. Many more examples also exist.

As you can guess, observing the body in this way and treating it from this perspective involves a lifetime of study. You can learn how to "zap" a muscle with an electrical stimulation machine to decrease a spasm on a week- end course. You can even get some techniques to begin to reverse a forward head posture. But what you cannot get is an understanding of the intricacies of the musculoskeletal and fascial systems until you know the whole system, and work with it. So be wary of what some practitioners may promise, and check credentials as best you can.

Almost all of the information just presented about TMJ holds true for headache. The practioners that you seek help from may feel that headaches are caused by certain factors. The way in which headaches get treated often depends on how the practitioners views the cause of headache. Typically headaches are treated as follows: drugs, dietary modification, **biofeedback**, relaxation exercises, evaluation for allergies or other systemic causes, and psychiatry. Symptomatic relief can be found from these methods, and occasional cures. Avoiding certain dietary irritants makes good sense. So does relaxation. But who wants to stay on medication indefinitely? There clearly needs to be a better alternative and there is!

What I have found is that often there is a structural or physical component to headache. One powerful factor contributing to a person developing headaches is, once again, the presence of a forward head posture. The importance of this finding cannot be overlooked. When the head gets tipped back on the neck, a great deal of pressure is put on pain sensitive structures. Compression of the suboccipital muscles and the greater occipetal nerve which pierces through them is thought to be one of the leading causes of headache. By realigning the head on the neck, so that it is in a more upright position, pressure on these sensitive structures is relieved. This is done through the various treatment techniques previously discussed.

Another common cause of headache is **fascial** tightness, which can develop anywhere within the **fascial** sheath of the body. **Fascial** tightness leads to restriction of tissue. When these restrictions are present, they can put pressure on any pain sensitive structure. These restrictions can occur anywhere and travel anywhere in the body throughout the **fascial** network, including the head. They can communicate into the **dural** system of the spine and head, thus distorting these tissues and causing headache. You may remember the picture of the cloth which was distorted by the pulled threads, in Chapter 4. The treatment modalities most effective in relieving these restrictions are twofold: **myofascial release** to relieve the peripheral restrictions, and **craniosacral therapy** to restore mobility to the deep central structures within the **craniosacral** system. By relieving these restrictions and by restoring more "play" within the entire **fascial** system, one's **physiological** adaptive range is restored. This means that the body will be able to withstand greater demands and adapt to the stresses placed upon it, because the tissues will have regained their length.

Another common cause of headache is lack of neck mobility, particularly of the upper two cervical vertebrae. Normal neck mobility is present when all seven of the cervical vertebrae are able to move through their full range of motion. Stiffness of the joints can lead to headache and face pain. This occurs in part because of the extensive nerve connections between the neck, the head, and the face. Proper functioning of the spinal nerves, which exit the spine at each vertebral level, can become impaired when the joints become tight. Because the neck is not moving normally, abnormal sensory information is being fed back to the **Central Nervous System**, which continues the pain/tightness cycle. Restoring neck mobility improves the overall functioning of the nerves and addresses one important factor in headache production.

All four of these major areas need to be identified and cleared in the management of headache. If a forward head posture is observed, it needs to be corrected. If the **craniosacral** system is in dysfuntion, it needs to be restored to proper functioning. If there are **fascial** restrictions, they need to be relieved. If the neck and overall spinal mobility is found to be poor, normal range of motion needs to be reestablished. I have found that when structural integrity is restored to those areas, headaches can rarely exist.

Western Medicine with all of its technology has so much to offer in the area of TMJ and headache. The refinement of diagnostic radiology gives us clearer pictures in which to view the body, the breakthroughs in the field of dentistry offer better, more comfortable alternatives to treatment, and the use of high technology treatment modalities makes the overall management of cases easier for the practitioner and more pleasing for the patient. And what is also true is that Western Medicine's greatest strength, its commitment to the scientific method, which has lead to so many discoveries, is also its greatest weakness. Utilization of the scientific method can be viewed as a strength of medicine, because treatment methods undergo testing to establish if they are valid and reliable. In this way, conducting experiments, which measure the effectiveness of treatment, function as a quality control. But by strictly adhering to the scientific method, modern medicine has greatly limited itself. It has done this by ignoring or discounting that which cannot be measured. Often, valuable, applicable information is missed because it fell between the lines of an experiment or in between the numbers on a statistical scale. The scientific method takes into account only what has statistically worked in the past for a majority of people. But this is not the whole story.

Dr. Bernie Siegel, in his book, Love, Medicine, and Miracles, says, "Science teaches us that we must see in order to believe, but we must also believe in order to see." He further goes on to say, "One generation's miracles may be another's scientific fact. Do not close your eyes to acts or events that are not always measureable. They happen by means of an inner energy available to all of us." When the science of medicine catches up with the art of medicine, it will become a stronger and more effective force.

There is a story of a man who is travelling in the Middle East. He is stopped by another man who raises a knife above his head and asks, "Are you a Moslem or a Christian?" The man thinks for a moment and answers, "I am a tourist." We are not all Moslems or Christian, and answering as such, trying to fit everyone into a system which does not account for variability, has cost us dearly.

There are many alternative methods of treatment, which could be considered on the fringe of Western Medicine, that can add a new dimension to your healing process. These are viable alternatives that work. And in fact, my profession is considered one such alternative. The practitioners of these techniques, generally, take great care in their work, and are often dedicated to a lifetime of learning. Many strive to live what they teach and practice. As with anything, there will be those individuals who will behave less than professionally. Shop well!

I will direct you to an excellent book called, Hands on Healing, which was compiled by the editors of Prevention Magazine. The leading proponents of the various alternative approaches present the basic philosophy of their technique and explain how the techniques are administered. I will list just some of the alternative healing approaches outlined in the book: Chiropractic, Acupressure, Alexander Technique, Applied Kinesiology, Aromatherapy, Aston-Patterning, Body Wraps, Deep Muscle Therapy, Esalen Massage, Feldenkrais Method, Hellerwork, Hydrotherapy, Lomilomi, Myotherapy, Naprapathy, Osteopathy, Polarity Therapy, Rolfing, Reflexology, and Trager Approach. What these disciplines have in common is that they work on the body in a particular manner, consistent with how the body is viewed in that system of thought. Many of the sections give information on how to locate practitioners in your area. If you are interested in learning about any of these alternative techniques, I would recommend that you read each section, see which methods interest you or make the most sense to you, find someone who practices that method, and see how your body responds to the work. Your body is its own internal laboratory. Let it decide!

After having experienced Chiropractic, Rolfing, Feldenkrais, Massage of all types, Reflexology, Deep Muscle Therapy, Craniosacral Therapy, Myofascial Release, and Acupuncture, (not all at the same time) what I can say is that as simple and trite as it may appear on paper, it has made my life better. It is not that my life is not good. But to accomplish what I want to accomplish, to achieve my full potential, I use these tools to give me an edge and maintain my direction. For many people, body work is considered regular maintenance for their body and good insurance. Think about it!

You will remember that we talked about that special place inside of you where only one person is allowed, yourself. In this space, you manage, sort, prioritize, think, feel, and all kinds of other things too numerous to list. This place is you. This is who you are. The extent to which you are aware of this private space, is the extent to which you are in control of your life. Making good friends with yourself on this level, exploring the inner workings of how you process events that happen to you in your life is the groundwork you need to do to "Know Thyself."

By paying attention to your random thoughts, you will begin to make conscious what was previously below the level of your consciousness. We call this our self-talk. Self-talk is the private conversation that we have with ourselves all during the day. Becoming aware of how you talk to yourself is the first step in being able to choose to think about something differently. Choosing to think about something differently can lead to you changing your feelings about it. Only by changing your feeling about something do you have a chance to change the event itself.

For example, let's say that you are on an airplane which lands in Chicago, and the connecting flight, which is to take you to your final destination, gets cancelled. Do you say to yourself, "the airline always does this," and leave Chicago two days later? Or, do you say to yourself, "there must be a reason why this is happening," get off the plane and call to book your own reservation out of Chicago that night? By choosing positive self-talk we keep negative emotions in check, which allows us to think clearly and act decisively.

If you find yourself stuck in a cycle of negative self- talk such as, "this is terrible," or "I can't do this," practice changing this to, "I can do this," "Yes, it's hard, but I can take it one step at a time." Our self-talk about an event causes us to have a feeling about it, which causes us to act a certain way. Through the awareness that we gain from paying attention to our self talk, we can change how we view situations so that we can change the situations themselves. By changing our self talk from negative to positive we move from a fixed state of consciousness to one in which there is movement and therefore a possibility for a solution. If we stay victims in our heads, we will remain victims in our lives. THERE IS ALWAYS A SOLUTION! That solution is within you.

Writing this book has been a joy. If it has found a home with you on your little book shelves to be taken out and perused, then we have both been enriched. My intent was to lead you to a place where you would understand about headaches and TMJ, and in that understanding, would gain clarity and vision for yourself. This book may have answered many of your questions. It has probably also contributed to you asking more. The final thought that I would like to leave you with is this:

Be patient toward all that is unsolved in your heart.

And try to love the questions themselves.

-Rainer Maria Rilke

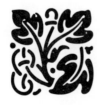

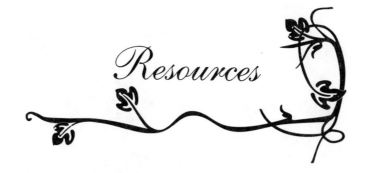

Resources

Glossary

Acupuncture: a Chinese method of treatment which views health and disease in terms of the balance or imbalance of energy in the body. The flow of energy, which is referred to as chi, is stimulated or diffused by inserting needles into points located on the skin.

Acupuncture point: a point on one of the energy lines or meridians of the body, according to Chinese Medicine. Stimulation of these points produce various body responses.

Acute: having severe symptoms and a short course.

Adrenalin: a substance which gets secreted into the system from the adrenal glands overlying the kidneys, which stimulates the body and triggers the flight/fight response.

Analgesic: a family of drugs, of which the primary physiological effect is pain relief.

Anti-depressant: a family of drugs, of which the primary physiological effect is mood elevation. A secondary effect may be pain relief.

Anti-inflammatory: a family of drugs, of which the primary physiological effect is reducing inflammation, which is the body's response to protect its tissues from injury or destruction.

Arthrogram: a picture of the inside of a joint, produced by taking an X-ray of a joint which has had dye injected into it. The presence of the dye in the joint makes possible the visualization of structures in the joint not visible by X-ray alone.

Arthroscope: a long needle-like instrument which is inserted into a joint. The scope is attached to a television monitor. Joint structures can be viewed, and certain surgical procedures can be performed through the arthroscope.

Arthroscopic Surgery: a procedure in which surgery is performed on a joint through a scope.

Articular Eminence: the most anterior portion of the temporal bone. The contacting surface of the condyle when the jaw is fully opened.

Beta blockers: a family of drugs, which blocks the transmission of impulses across certain nerve junctions thereby leading to decreased pain sensation. These drugs are suggested to be useful in treating headaches.

Biofeedback: a treatment technique, which utilizes a machine to give feedback to a subject on a particular body function, so that the body's response can then be modified. An example of this is electromyographic biofeedback which allows the function of muscle tension to be altered.

Bonding: a dental procedure in which a tooth can be built up or reshaped by applying a material that bonds to the tooth, matching both the color and texture.

Braces: a fixed appliance, which is attached to the teeth, for the purpose of changing their position.

Bruxism: clenching and grinding of the teeth.

Capping: a procedure in dentistry, where a crown in applied to a tooth. If a tooth has deteriorated, and enough of the tooth is intact, a crown of metal, porcelain, or gold can be applied.

Capsule: the enclosing structure of a joint comprised of connective tissue. The capsule unites the ends of bones.

Cartilage: the white elastic substance which covers the surfaces of bone and forms part of the bony skeleton.

Cavity: an area of decay within a tooth. When left untreated a destructive process ensues leading to decalcification of the tooth enamel.

Central Nervous System (CNS): the brain, spinal cord and nerve roots. The main relay and regulating system for the entire body.

Chronic: persisting for a long time, at least three months, showing little change or slow progress.

Cold therapy: the therapeutic use of cold, usually in the form of cold packs or vapocoolant sprays.

Coefficient of friction: a number, indicating the amount of resistance to movement inherent in a substance. The lower the number the slicker the substance due to its tendency to cause less friction.

Condyle: the rounded end of a bone, e.g. the condyle of the mandible.

Connective tissue: specialized tissue such as ligaments and tendons that connect various body parts.

Counterirritation effect: superficial irritation with the intention of relieving some other irritation, e.g. ice application to relieve pain.

Craniosacral therapy (CST): techniques which restore regular rhythmic movement to the cranial/sacral system which is primarily composed of the dura (the deep fascia). The dura is attached to the sutures of the cranium and the entire spinal canal, ending at the sacral bone at the end of the spine.

Cranium: the head

Crepitus: a crackling noise produced by the joint upon movement.

CT scan: computed tomography. Images of slices of tissue arrived at when a body part is scanned by a CT tube. This image is more accurate than a standard X-ray.

Diaphragm: the strong, dome-shaped sheet of muscle, which separates the thoracic and abdominal cavities of the body. It is the primary muscle of breathing.

Disc: a cartilagenous cushion within a joint.

Dislocation: a situation where joint surfaces become completely or partially separated, thus straining surrounding joint tissues.

Dura: the outermost covering of the brain and spinal cord which is composed of connective tissue.

Dysfunction: abnormal or imperfect action or functioning, e.g. a dysfunctional TMJ is one which will not open to normal.

Electrical stimulation: the fundamental quantity in nature consisting of electrons and positron particles. This can be applied to the body to produce therapeutic effects.

Electroacupuncture device: a machine designed to deliver an electrical stimulus to acupuncture points.

Fascia: a connective tissue network coursing three dimensionally through the entire body.

Flight/Fight Response: a method of protection, a primitive response of the body, where adrenalin is pumped into the system in order to prepare a person to run from danger or defend himself.

Flouroscopy: examination of a body part by means of a flouroscope, which displays a moving picture on a flourescent screen. This is refered to as a dynamic radiograph, where the actual opening and closing motions of the TMJ can be observed.

Fossa: a pit or depression in a bone, e.g. the fossa of the temporal bone.

Freeway space: the space created between the top and bottom teeth when the tongue is in its resting position.

Gingivitis: inflammation of the gums, which is the fleshy structure covering the tooth bearing border of the jaw.

Gliding: a sliding of the joint surfaces which occurs within a joint upon movement. This occurs in the TMJ in the phase of opening.

Gouty arthritis: deterioration and inflammation of a joint due to gout, which is a disturbance of the purine metabolism of the body.

Hinge joint: a type of joint allowing primarily for the motions of opening and closing, e.g. the TMJ.

Hygiene: cleaning habits such as brushing the teeth, flossing, and regular cleaning of the teeth by the dentist.

Hypoglycemia: a deficiency of sugar in the blood.

Hypothyroidism: a deficiency of thyroxin which is produced by the thyroid gland, leading to a lowered metabolic rate.

Internal derrangement: a mechanical problem within a joint, e.g. anterior displacement of the disc within the TMJ.

Iontophoresis: a procedure in which electrical stimulation is used to drive a drug through the skin, thus enhancing circulation and healing.

Isometric contraction: a muscular contraction in which the muscles generate force, but there is no observable movement of the joint across which the muscles are contracting, e.g. rhythmic stabilization of the TMJ.

Joint mobilization techniques: manual techniques which restore normal joint motion.

Kinetic Chain: a flexible series of joined links, such as the vertebra of the spine, where a change in the movement at one segment, influences the movement at the other segments. Another example of a kinetic chain is a string of dominoes falling.

Kreb Cycle: the metabolic process, which occurs within muscle, and creates most of the energy the body uses for its many functions.

Laser: light amplification by stimulated emission of radiation. An extremely intense, small, focused beam of light with all of the light waves in phase.

Lateral pterygoid muscle: a muscle which closes the jaw. It attaches to the front of the disc.

Ligaments: a tough band of connective tissue connecting bones or supporting organs.

Malocclusion: abnormal contact of the teeth.

Mandible: the lower jaw.

Masseter muscle: a muscle, which closes the jaw and is located superficially in the cheek.

Medial pterygoid muscle: a muscle, which closes the jaw and is located deep in the cheek.

Menisectomy: removal of the meniscus or disc from a joint.

Moist heat packs: hydrocolator packs, which deliver a penetrating moist heat to the body, in order to stimulate circulation, promote healing, and enhance relaxation.

MRI Magnetic Resonance Imaging: An imaging modality which utilizes magnetic energy rather than X-ray to produce its image. The picture produced displays the body part in great anatomic detail.

Muscle relaxant: a family of drugs, in which the primary physiological effect is relaxation of the muscle. A secondary effect may be anxiety reduction.

Muscle spasm: an involuntary tightening or shortening of a muscle.

MPD Myofascial Pain Dysfunction: An abnormal state of the musculature and its fascia leading to improper functioning of the part. A leading cause of TMJ.

Myofascial release techniques: manual procedures designed to specifically affect the fascia of the body by releasing the restrictions that form three dimensionally due to trauma or inflammation, thus restoring the muscular, and fascial system to normal.

Noninvasive therapy: the application of techniques which do not alter the body permanently. A conservative approach, e.g. removal of teeth would be considered invasive therapy, while most all of physical therapy is noninvasive.

Occipetal nerve: a nerve which pierces through the muscles of the upper neck, and can become compressed by a spasm of these muscles. Irritation of this nerve is a common cause of headache.

Occlusion: the contact of the teeth between the upper and lower jaw.

Organic disease: a pathological condition, involving one of the many systems of the body, such as circulatory or immune, which requires medical attention.

Orthodontics: the art and science of changing the position of the teeth, in order to secure and stabilize the occlusion.

Orthognathic surgery: surgery to correct defects in the bones of the jaw.

Overbite: the extension of the upper anterior teeth over the lower anterior teeth when the jaw is closed.

Pathologies: diseases

Periodontal disease: disease of gum tissue, which can lead to deterioration of the jaw bone.

Phonophoresis: a procedure in which ultrasound is used to drive a drug through the skin to enhance circulations and promote healing.

Physical agent: a therapeutic modality such as heat, cold, electrical stimulation, laser, or ultrasound.

Physiological: function. Functional mechanisms underlying the life processes. Anatomy is the study of structure. Physiology is the study of function.

Plain film: a standard X-ray.

Postural plumb line: a string with a weight on the end which forms a vertical line in gravity. The person stands in back of the vertical line while being evaluated. This is a standard tool used to evaluate how far one deviates from the ideal vertical.

Prognathic: a protruding forward of the lower jaw.

Pulp chamber: the body of a tooth.

Radiographs: the taking of pictures of internal structures of the body by exposure of specially sensitized film to X-rays.

Repositioning splint: an appliance which alters the position of the lower jaw, either forward or to one side.

Resting splint: an appliance which separates the teeth, gently stretching the TMJ, and promoting relaxation of the jaw muscles.

Retrognathic: a moving backward of the lower jaw.

Rolling: a spin of the moving joint surface (the mandible) which occurs within the joint upon movement. Rolling of the TMJ occurs in the first phase of opening.

Root canal: the channels under each tooth which house the nerves.

Silastic disc: type of implant commonly used to replace a torn or worn disc.

Splint: an appliance, usually made of a tough acrylic resin.

Spray and stretch: a form of cold therapy where a vapocoolant substance is sprayed across the entire length of a muscle while the muscle is in its fully stretched position. The purpose of this technique is to release the restrictions within the fascia of the muscle.

Subacute: somewhat acute, between acute and chronic.

Sutures: the line of union of adjoining bones of the skull.

Synovial fluid: the transparent, viscous fluid produced by the synovial membrane, which is found in joint cavities, bursae, and tendon sheaths. It is the lubricating fluid of joints.

Synovial membrane: a thin layer of tissue on the underside of the joint capsule which produces synovial fluid.

Temporal bone: the bone which comprises the temple and contains the fossa of the TMJ.

Temporalis muscle: a muscle, which closes the jaw and is located in the temple area of the head.

Tendons: a fibrous cord of connective tissue continuous with the fibers of a muscle, which attaches muscle to bone or cartilage.

TENS Transcutaneous Electrical Nerve Stimulation: Electrical stimulation which travels across the skin from electrode to electrode, is usually applied by means of a portable stimulator, and is used for its counterirriation effects, to reduce inflammation and promote healing.

Tinnitis: a noise in the ears, which may at times be heard by others beside the patient.

Tomogram: an X-ray of a section of tissue making it more accurate than a standard X-ray. Computed tomography.

Trigger point: a hyperirritable focus in a muscle which is often present in taut bands within a muscle.

Ultrasound: mechanical radiant energy above the frequency which can normally be heard. The body absorbs the sound waves and converts the sound energy to heat, thereby increasing circulation and promoting healing.

Viscosity: that quality of fluid which describes its flow characteristics, e.g. water has a low viscosity while honey has a high viscosity. Synovial fluid is highly viscous.

Whiplash: a situation in which a force applied to the body causes it to be whipped first in one direction, and then in the opposite direction, e.g. what happens to the neck in a rear end collision.

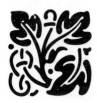

Bibliography

Benson, Herbert. Your Maximum Mind. Random House, New York. 1987.

Benson, Herbert. The Relaxation Response. Avon Books, New York. 1967.

Borysenko, Joan. Minding the Body/Mending the Mind. Bantam New Age Books, New York. 1984.

Dyer, Wayne. Your Erroneous Zones. Avon Books, New York. 1976.

Feltman, John, ed., Hands on Healing. Rodale Press, Emmaus, Pennsylvania. 1988.

Gawain, Shakti. Creative Visualization. Whatever Publishing Inc., San Rafael. 1978.

Ott, John. Health and Light. Pocket Books, New York. 1973.

Peck, Scott. The Road Less Traveled. Simon and Schuster, New York. 1978.

Prudden, Bonnie. Pain Erasure. Ballantine Books, New York. 1980.

Schneider, Mark and Meyer, Ellen. What to Do When You're Feeling Blue. Contemporary Books, Chicago. 1989.

Siegel, Bernard. Love, Medicine, and Miracles. Harper and Row, New York. 1986.

Siegel, Bernard. Peace, Love, and Healing. Harper and Row, New York. 1989.

Smith, Gerald. Headaches Aren't Forever. Newtown, 1987.

Travell, Janet G. Myofascial Pain and Dysfunction. Williams and Wilkins, Baltimore. 1983. (MEDICAL TEXTBOOK)

Upledger, John. Craniosacral Therapy. Eastland Press, Chicago. 1983. (MEDICAL TEXTBOOK)

Viorst, Judith. Necessary Losses. Simon and Schuster, New York. 1986.

Wilson, Randy, ed., The Non-Chew Cookbook. Wilson Publishing, Box 2190, Glenwook Springs, CO 81602.

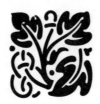

Index

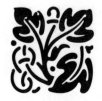